THE INTERMITTENT FASTING:

How to Live Fit, Lose Weight fast

and Stay Young

Inspiring Beginner's Guide with

Motivation Lists, Action Plans,

Progress Chart

and Weight Loss Tracker

By

Olivia A. Stone

Only I can Change my Life, no One Can Do It for Me

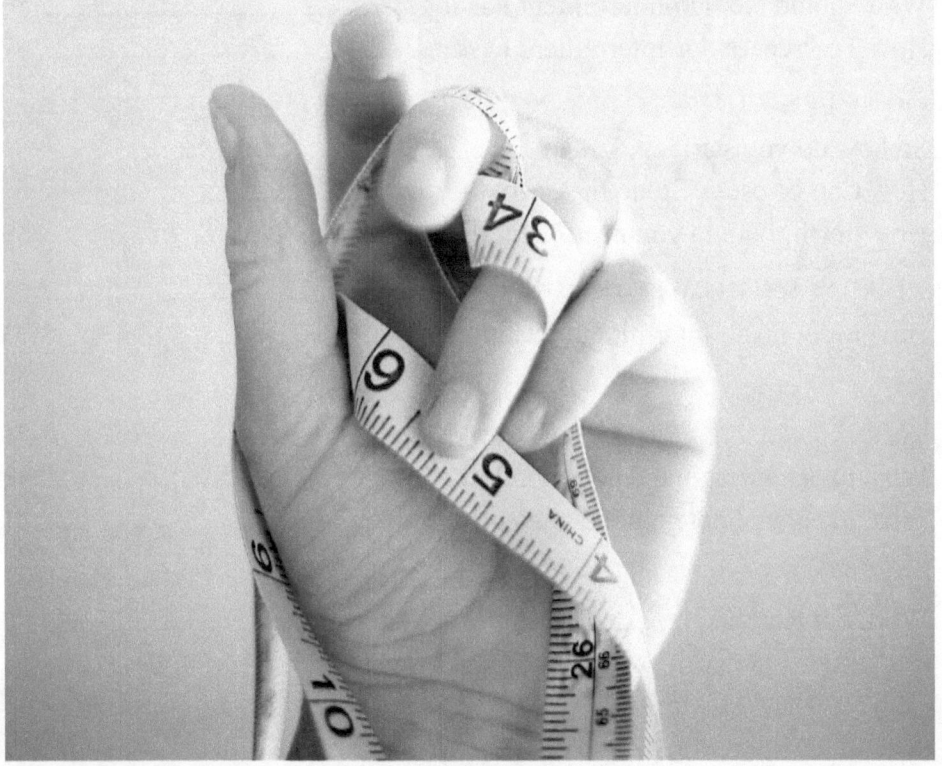

TABLE OF CONTENTS

INTRODUCTION

There is a massive problem in the world today when it comes to health. That major problem I'm speaking about is nutrition. Everything is so messed up because the corporations and manufacturers BECAUSE they need YOU and ME to buy products that can be produced for profits. Everyone, and this includes me, gets so confused on topics like this, when they have to read 100 different experts, say a 100 different things.

This book contains inspiring quotes, motivation lists, action plans, progress chart and weight loss tracker for readers.

This made me remember when I was about to lose my weight, I picked up this great book which has opened my eyes to probably the oldest new concept for fat loss. The book is called Eat Stop Eat by Brad Pillon and in a nutshell, it is about intermittent fasting.

So I assign a weekend I am going to try my first 24 hours planned fast. Basically this means I will be going without food for 24 hours between dinner last night and dinner tonight. There is a lot of uncertainty with what I am doing simply because I have never done this before.

As with my training ideas, you will know that simple doesn't always, well rarely, means easy. I expect the same to come of this. So sit back, relax and lets see what happens!

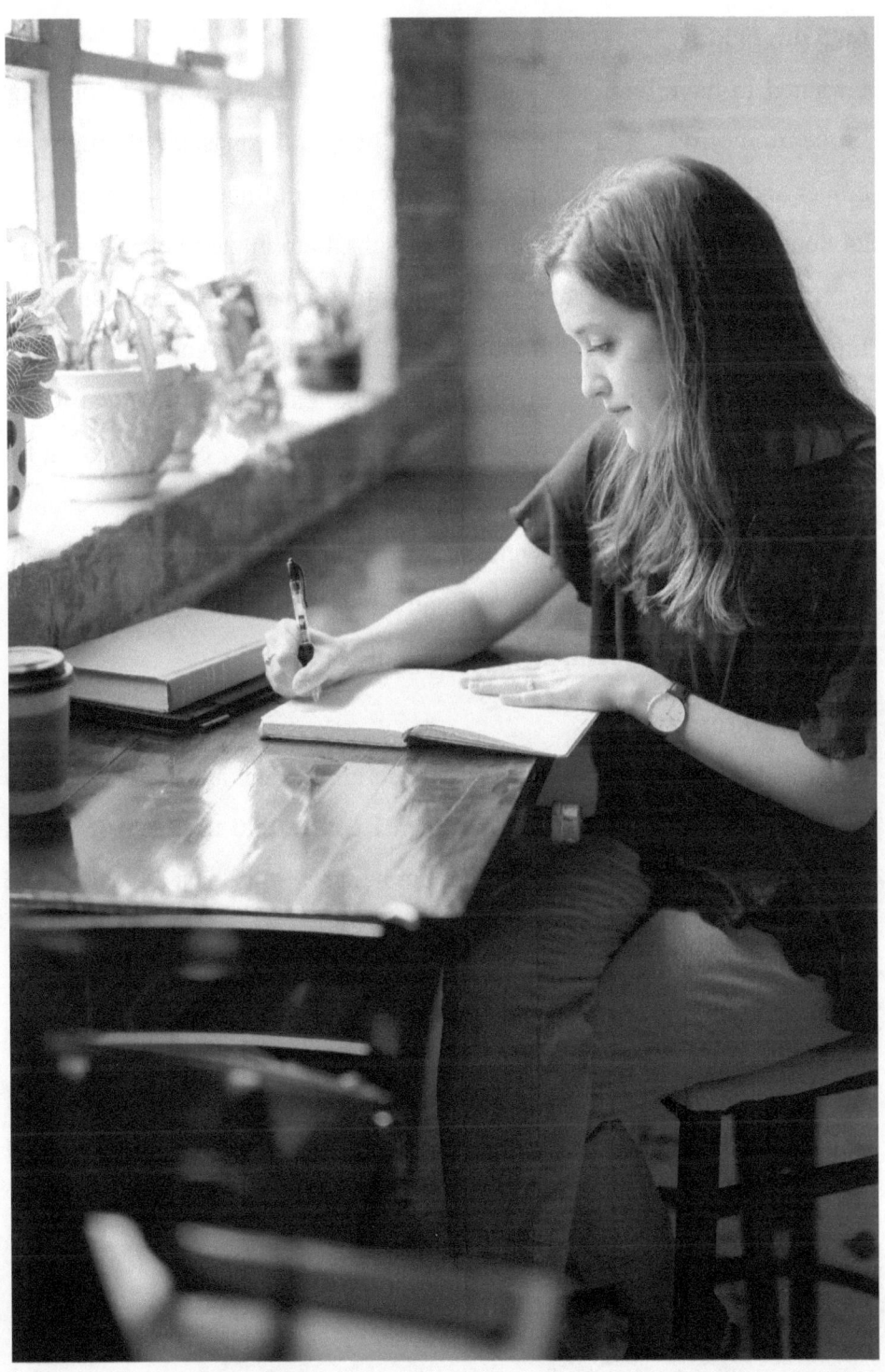

6:45 pm Friday

I wanted to have dinner as early as possible tonight, so that I could eat sooner tomorrow. That didn't happen though. I smashed through my dinner and probably ate too much in anticipation of not eating for another 24 hours. Then I have my first 'food' thought. I am in the kitchen making a cup of tea and went to grab some food off the dinner plate that hadn't been finished. Whoops, I can't eat that. But I don't actually want to eat it; I am stuffed like a pig. But it is there and I felt like eating it. I didn't eat it, but all I can think about, for now, is food and the fact that I can't be eating for the next 23 hours and 48 minutes!

After playing the Wii for a while it is time for bed, and I haven't thought of food or felt hungry again. Normally I would have something to eat before bed but not tonight, no big deal really.

8:07 am Saturday

I was lucky enough to get a sleep this morning. Rach and Ash were up a bit earlier, but I was catching Zs. When I got up, I'm thinking of what I can't have for breakfast, although I'm not hungry. So it's just a black coffee and that's fine. Everything seems normal, plenty of energy, no jitters or shakes or anything different to be honest.

10:23 am Saturday

About to head into town to see a friend in the hospital. Just had coffee and water today. Thoughts of food are far away, although I suspect that will change when we pass all of the food outlets and Rach and Ash have lunch.

1.14 pm Saturday

We have been somewhat busy this morning and the time has gone quite quickly. It isn't until I look at the clock and realize how late it is (compared to what I would have normally eaten by now). Rach and Ash are getting into some corn chips as we wait in the car at my mom's house. I would have said I'm hungry but I wasn't before the chips came out and I started salivating! So am I really hungry or do I just want food? I'd suggest it's the latter as I don't care to eat anything else once I have had a green tea and black coffee.

I am starting to think that dinner time will come around quickly now and the 24 hours will have passed without any bother. It's strange because I normally feel 'hungry' if I have a late breakfast.

4.19 pm Saturday

The girls are asleep, and I have had a quick 20-minute recharging nap. I would probably do this three times per week depending on how I feel. So it has nothing to do with my energy levels because of the fasting. I feel completely normal (well as normal as I have ever felt!!)

I can't believe there is only just over two hours to go. I must admit that I have been thinking about what I will be eating for dinner tonight quite regularly, but that is fairly common for me.

6:02 pm Saturday

has passed me by. The girls are still asleep!! So, I might get a start on dinner. Some meat and vegetables should do the trick.I've been working on the website and doing some research for my bootcamp launch and the time.

7:01 pm Saturday

Well, the 24 hours has been and gone, and I am amazed at how simple (and easy) that was. I was a bit scared of the unknown last night because I hadn't done anything like this before. Now I think it has to be the easiest weight loss solution going around. I feel as though I could go for longer as well. Now that I can eat there isn't an overwhelming feeling that I need to stuff my face because I am hungry.

I don't know what real hunger feels like anymore. I haven't eaten in over 24 hours, yet I don't feel compelled to eat. Strange, I know, but very hard to explain.

Because my energy levels were so good I want to try a 24 hour fast during the work week and throw in a training session as well. That will be a bigger test but after the ease of this phase, I can't see why that would be any more difficult.

The Intermittent Fasting: How to Live Fit, Lose Weight fast and Stay Young. Inspiring Beginner's Guide is also the best book for you when you want to lose weight and live a healthy life.

This book majorly focus on how to take action, the information and how-to's should have actionable tips that they can take away from the book But for you to have the actionable tips is not enough but also knowing how to use this book for fast turn around of your goals in other to achieve.

As Les Brown once said that if you set goals and go after them with all the determination you can muster, your gifts will take you places that will amaze you.Setting a goal Is half way success of achieving your aim but you have to go after .

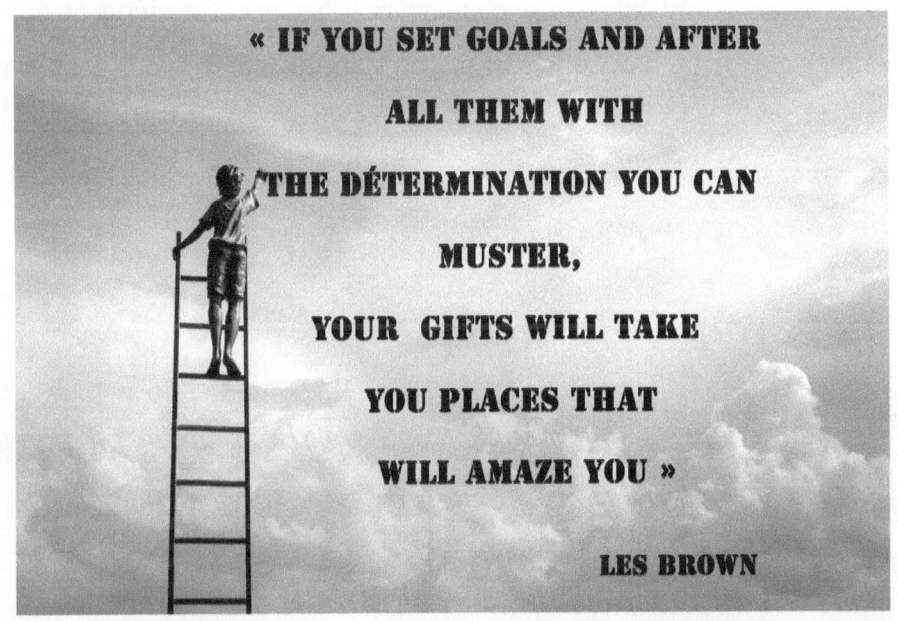

« IF YOU SET GOALS AND AFTER
ALL THEM WITH
THE DÉTERMINATION YOU CAN
MUSTER,
YOUR GIFTS WILL TAKE
YOU PLACES THAT
WILL AMAZE YOU »

LES BROWN

In a world cluttered with to-do-list makers and new-year-resolution breakers, the temptation for all of us, is to bite off more than we can chew. We first spent money buying stationery, which we then promptly fill up with unending lists of to-dos. What we don't do is know 'How to achieve your goals' and therefore end up frustrated and defeated.

Goal-setting can be an emotional high, but, to ensure our to-do lists see the light of the day, we need plans and the ability to stick to them. While each of us is as different as the goals we hope to accomplish, here are a few common pointers on going about this simple task that is often the topic of much discussion. Now, having said all that, the first thing you need to do is to get the stationery out. For people who have a passion for stationery, buying colorful index cards, might help. Then, figure out the goal in your mind. What is it exactly that you want to achieve - finish the book you started to Lose five kilos in two months? Whatever it is, write it down clearly. Next, write down the reason you want to achieve your goal. This serves as a reminder and a motivation to have it accomplished. This could be the first step in helping you figure out for yourself, how to achieve your goals by making plans that work for you.

What's your WHY?

Take a moment to write some contemplations down on paper. What's your motivation to choosing an Intermittent Fasting lifestyle?

_____

_____

_____

_____

_____

_____

_____

_____

On the Road to the Better Health

If   I   Make   Small   Daily   Changes   I   Will

_____
_____
_____
_____
_____
_____
_____
_____
_____

Who Else Can I Positively Impact With My Changes ?

_____
_____
_____
_____
_____
_____
_____
_____
_____
_____
_____
_____
_____
_____
_____
_____

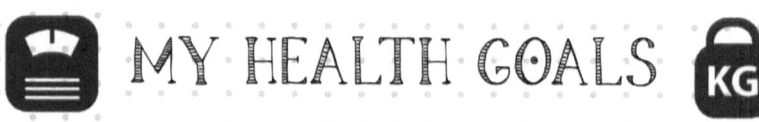

MY HEALTH GOALS

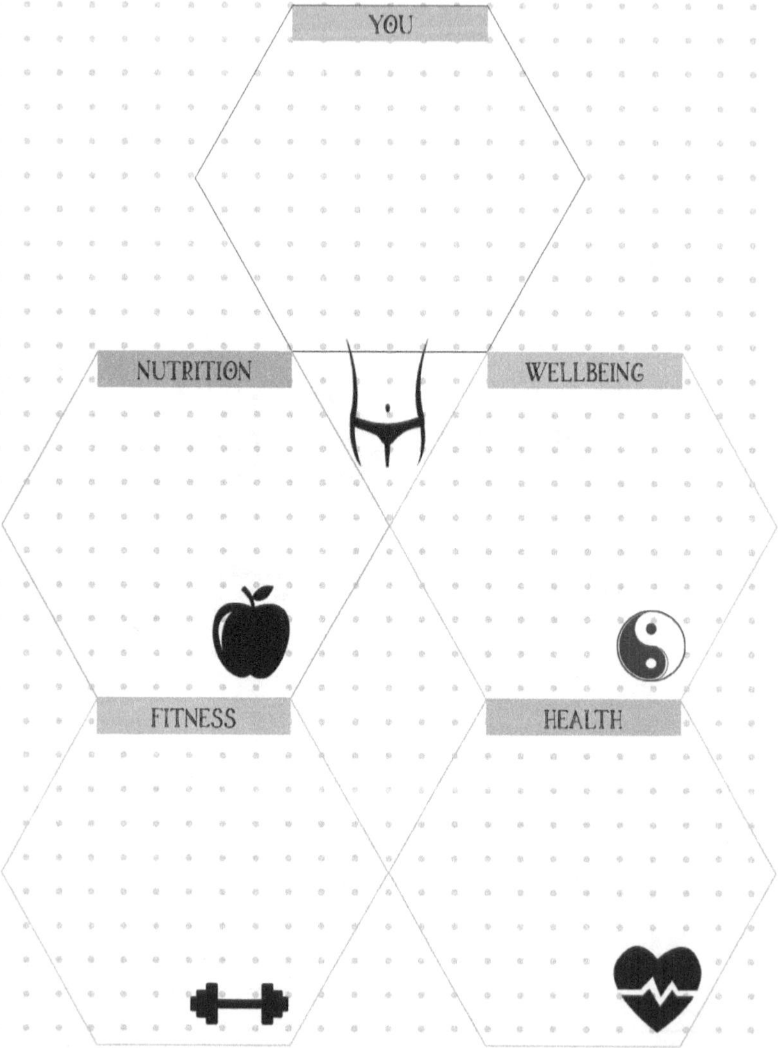

YOU

NUTRITION

WELLBEING

FITNESS

HEALTH

Find a time during the day or at night, when you will be able to work toward achieving your goal. It could be in the wee hours of the morning, if you need quiet time to write. Or when the kids are in school, if you'd like to run on the treadmill without interruption.

_____

_____

_____

_____

_____

_____

_____

_____

_____

_____

_____

_____

_____

_____

_____

_____

_____

_____

_____

_____

_____

A Goal Without A Plan Is Just A Wish

Once you're done with your list and action plan, waste no time in getting started. About a week later, review your progress. Are the timings really working for you? Have you been productive? If not, don't beat yourself up about it. One of the best ways to achieve your goals, is to evaluate your progress midway and fix anything that's not working. Change the time, alter the plan but don't give up.

Remember to visualize the outcome. If the goal you want to achieve is dropping five kilos, then see yourself fitting into clothes that you can't fit into, now. If the goal is to become a best-selling children's author, picture yourself receiving awards, talking to the press and giving guest speeches. It's an established truth that if you cannot see yourself accomplishing what you set out to do, chances are, you won't accomplish it.

And finally, remember that no one can tell you how to achieve your goals. Goals and the process of achieving them are as unique as the people who make them. After reading all the material on the subject, you are alone with your to-do list. Only you know your passion, what drives you and what it takes to achieve your goals.

Use that knowledge well.

CHAPTER 1
WHAT IS INTERMITTENT FASTING ?

I t is an eating pattern where one fasts for a set period of time and then eats for another set period of time. The three most common approaches that I have seen in the literature are the once a week/month, 24 hours and the daily 16/8 or 20/4 intermittent fast. During the 24 hours routine, the individual doesn't eat or drink anything with the exception of water, green or black tea for a 24-hour period. Then, after that 24 hour period has expired they begin eating again. During the 16/8 or 20/4 routine, the individual does not eat for either 16 to 20 hours and then eats meals during the other four to eight hour period.

The question of whether an intermittent fast is healthy or not is still undecided, and that is why you should consult your physician when wanting to alter your diet in a manner such as this.

Will I lose weight doing an intermittent fast? This is also a very debatable question, because it really depends on many other mitigating factors such as, what is your "normal" non-fasting diet consisting of, do you have any underlying medical issues etc... If you fast for one day, but your diet consists of nothing but processed foods, fast food, animal products and desserts then no, your probably not going to lose weight. One must have a sound base of nutritional knowledge before they can use intermittent fasting as a weight loss system.

Generally, this type of eating/fasting routine has been widely used by athletes, weight lifters and body builders as a way to "lean out" and decrease their body fat percentage. Those three groups all have one thing in common...

They all understand the nuts and bolts of nutrition as well as the more advanced aspects of nutrition, so adding in something like the routines discussed above to lose a few percentage points off of their body fat and "lean out" is an easy addition to their routine.

Intermittent fasting weight loss is one of the most effective ways to shed off your extra pounds. The ideas on intermittent fasting weight loss challenge most of the previously held beliefs on losing. Those who are seeking new ways to lose weight effectively have quickly embraced its ideas.

What is IF Weight Loss?

Let me start by clarifying that intermittent fasting is not a diet. You are probably tired of trying anything with the word 'diet' on it when it comes to weight loss. Intermittent fasting is a way of eating that involves a structured program on the times you eat and when you do not eat. You structure your program according to your taste. If you can handle it, fast for a whole day! I recommend that you fast for 12 full hours before eating. You can increase your fasting period later as you continue with the program.

What Makes it Different?

You probably have tried diets such as Atkins diet based on the frequent feeding theory if you have tried to lose weight. Simply, proponents of such diets told you to eat often during the day. The idea was that the more you eat, the faster your metabolism. The faster your metabolism, the more fat you will lose. Of course, you do know that the more you eat, the more you wanted to eat and the more your weight remained. When you are on an intermittent program, you will have to cut down your meal frequency. Sometimes, you have to do without breakfast.

Tell Me More

You probably sleep for around six to eight hours. During this time, your body is in fasting mode. When your body is in fasting mode, it usually produces more insulin. More insulin in your body causes your body to have increased insulin sensitivity. When your body has increased insulin sensitivity, you lose more fat. The brilliance of intermittent fasting weight loss program is that you skip breakfast to extend the period of your body's insulin sensitivity. This means that your body is going to be on fat loss mode for a longer period. You will lose more weight.

A longer fasting mode also has a good effect on the growth hormone levels in your body. By skipping breakfast or eating during a specific period, your body produces growth hormone. Growth hormone is what you want your body producing when you are trying to lose weight. This is simply because; growth hormone promotes weight loss in your body. When you are on an intermittent fasting weight loss program, your growth hormone levels are usually at their peak. You will be your more weight during this period. High Growth hormone levels in simply body also have several other health benefits. This program is losing amazing!

INTERMITTENT FASTING SYSTEM

The lifestyle you follow during Intermittent Fasting will be determined by the results that you are looking for and where you are starting out from as well, so take a look at yourself and ask the question what do I want from this?

Although there are several ways you can do intermittent fasting we are only going to look at the 24 hours fasting system which is what I used to lose 27 pounds over two months. The basic method is to fast twice a week for 24 hours, it makes sense to do this a few days apart and it is easier if you pick a day when you are busy so that you do not become distracted by feelings of hunger. Initially you may feel some hunger pangs but these will pass, and as you become more accustomed to intermittent fasting, you may find as I have that feelings of hunger no longer present you with a problem. You may find that you have great focus and concentration while fasting which is the opposite of what you would expect but many people experience this.

There are many benefits to intermittent fasting which you will notice as you progress, some of these benefits include more energy, less bloating, a clearer mind and a general

feeling of wellness. It's important not to succumb to any temptation to binge eat after a fasting period as this will negate the effect gained from the intermittent fasting period.

So, in conclusion, just by following a 24 hours intermittent fasting plan twice a week for a few weeks, you will lose weight but if you can improve your diet on the days that you don't fast then you will lose more weight and if you can stick to this system then you will keep the weight off without resorting to any crash diets or diets that are just impossible to stick to.

Intermittent Fasting For Women

Intermittent fasting is also known as alternate-day fasting, although there are certainly some variations on this diet. The American Journal of Clinical Nutrition performed a study recently that enrolled 16 obese men and women on a 10-week program. On the fasting days, participants consumed food to 25% of their estimated energy needs. The rest of the time, they received dietary counseling but were not given a specific guideline to follow during this time.

As expected, the participants lost weight due to this study, but what researchers really found interesting were some specific changes. The subjects were all still obese after just ten weeks, but they had shown improvement in cholesterol, LDL-cholesterol, triglycerides, and systolic blood pressure. What made this an interesting find was that most people have to lose more weight than these study participants before seeing the same changes. It was a fascinating find which has spurred a great number of people to try fasting. Intermittent fasting for women have some beneficial effects. What makes it important for women who are trying to lose weight is that women have a much higher fat proportion in their bodies. When trying to lose weight, the body primarily burns through carbohydrate stores with the first six hours and then starts to burn fat. Women who are following a healthy diet and exercise plan, may be struggling with stubborn fat, but fasting is a realistic solution to this.

Intermittent Fasting For Women Over 50

Obviously, our bodies and our metabolism changes when we hit menopause. One of the biggest changes that women over 50 experience is that they have a slower metabolism and they start to put on weight. Fasting may be a good way to reverse and prevent this weight gain though. Studies have shown that this fasting pattern helps to regulate appetite, and people who follow it regularly do not experience the same cravings that others do. If you're over 50 and trying to adjust to your slower metabolism, intermittent fasting can help you to avoid eating too much on a daily basis.

When you reach 50, your body also starts to develop some chronic diseases such as high cholesterol and high blood pressure. Intermittent fasting has been shown to decrease both cholesterol and blood pressure, even without a great deal of weight loss. If you've started to notice your numbers rising at the doctor's office each year, you may be able to bring them back down with fasting, even without losing much weight.

Intermittent fasting may not be a great idea for every woman. Anyone with a specific health condition or who tends to be hypoglycemic should consult with a doctor. However, this new dietary trend has specific benefits for women who naturally store more fat in their bodies and may have trouble getting rid of these fat stores.

Intermittent Fasting For Weight Loss Tips

There's no doubt about it that many people today are using intermittent fasting for weight loss. If you're not sure what intermittent fasting is it's when you strategically use periods of fasting to force your body into burning fat as a fuel source. This method of weight loss is highly effective but you have to make sure you're doing it right or else you can actually slow your metabolism.

While you are going through a fasting period, you should only be consuming water along with Branched Chain Amino Acids (BCAA) which will help prevent the breakdown of muscle. This may be too intense for some people because you will most likely experience hunger and there will be a high level of discipline necessary for intermittent fasting.

Those who are for this type of weight loss claim that they can get results quicker than traditional dieting practices such as calorie restriction.

If you're new to intermittent fasting then it's recommended that you do a trial period of 24 hours to make sure you can continue with doing these for an extended period of time. It's going to be natural to become easily irritable towards people during your fasting day so prepare for the worst. I prefer to have a cheat day prior to the fasting day so I can prepare my body for the fast and also accelerate the results. The massive caloric intake of the cheat day primes my body to burn more fat as a fuel source on the fasting day.

I also personally prefer to use Sundays as my fasting days because I have the least amount of interaction with society because once again it's very easy to become irritable. Be sure to take your BCAA's throughout the day in 5-10 gram servings like you would in place for regular meals. Eventually, after you have successfully completed the 24 hours fasts you can progress to more advanced methods of intermittent fasting such as using multiple ones throughout the week.

Intermittent fasting isn't going to be for everyone but if you're serious about getting some real results then this will definitely boost them. Everyone should still learn the basics of a healthy diet and exercise program. You can definitely workout on your fasting days to enhance the fat loss but it will be extremely difficult for many to muster the energy to do so. Overall just make sure you plan ahead prior to your fasting day as it will be instrumental in your success with the program.

Intermittent fasting, as described today, is one of the cheapest fasting diets to lose weight. It doesn't require any other tools such as pills or medicines, nor does it entail any expensive gym equipment. All it simply asks is a strict and stern discipline to fasting. Intermittent fasting, by definition connotes the regulation of food intake by not ingesting anything between major meals. Also, by the word intermittent, it follows that a sequential order of eating pattern must be attained.

There's a presumption among experts that the basis on how intermittent fasting actually works can be explained by reason of anatomy and physiology; or the study of the organ and organ systems in relation to their functions within our bodies. As explained by specialists such as physicians, within our brain stem lies the seat of satiety, hunger and thirst called the hypothalamus. The hypothalamus is a complex, multifarious organ which actually orders our body when to feel the urge to gobble.

Hence, should there be any desire for man to drink or eat; the hypothalamus is the one responsible for such action. Thus, if left untrained and left to do on its own will, satiety and hunger will increase to huge proportions.

Once this happens, the urge to drink or eat will also be magnified. Of course, there is no danger or risk to eating. There is absolutely nothing wrong with that; however, the quality of the food intake we eat also determines the state of health among individuals.

Likewise, if a person continually ingests foods that are not nutritious, say the one we see in fast foods or cafeterias; and done in large amounts, health is affected. Uncontrolled eating can lead to a host of diseases such as diabetes, hypertension, cardiac or heart problems and obesity.

The best way to start your fasting is to carefully plan your meals. Intermittent fasting works best if it is done regularly and habitually. This form of fasting diet to lose weight must be done in accordance with the willingness of the participant; and must be disciplined in order to achieve the desired effects. Aside from fasting, if you plan to lose weight, the amount of caloric intake must also be considered. So, aside from carefully planning the intermittent meals, the amount of calories must also be taken into consideration. Combining the two strategies will not just make you slim; it will help you get the weight you've always wanted. Moreover, training your hypothalamus to eat intermittently will have a huge impact on your urge to eat or drink which would lead to restraining your unhealthy eating habits.

Intermittent Fasting Vs Low Carb Diet?

If you are looking for a way to reduce your body fat, going low carb is one of the popular diet choices. There a number of different versions of low carb diets, from the famous Atkins diet to The South Beach Diet. Low Carb Diets are not new, the concept was not invented by Dr. Robert Atkins as many people seem to think. Low Carb diets even precede other US diet doctors such as Herman Tarnower and Herman Taller. Dieting Plans allowing you to eat meat, some dairy foods, salad and non-starchy vegetables, while restricting or banning foods containing sugar or starch were first promoted in the early 19th century by Jean Anthelme Brillat-Savarin. To this day the debate continues among Doctors and Nutritionists as to what is the best diet for us to follow and lose weight.

There is certainly evidence to show that initial weight loss while following a low carb diet does reduce body fat. In a recent study of popular diets (Gardner CD, Kiazand A, Alhassan S, et al. Comparison of the Atkins, Zone, Ornish, and LEARN diets for change in weight and related risk factors among overweight premenopausal women: the A TO Z Weight Loss Study: a randomized trial. JAMA 2007;297:969-77) The Atkins diet showed the best weight loss results over both a two month and a six-months period. This is the information you seen mentioned in the media on a regular basis. However over a 12 month period the Atkins diet results were not so impressive, and was no more effective than the other diets in the study. My own view based on my experience of trying low carb dieting is though effective in the short term, diets such as Atkins are not practical to follow in the long term. In my opinion, to lose body fat and control weight, the way we eat has to be possible to follow for the long term, not just for a few weeks. I have in the past done Atkins, The South Beach Diet, and Fat Flush. I have taken things from all of these diet plans, I use them as part of lifestyle today.

I also have a greater understanding of the effect refined carbohydrates have on my body, but the simple fact remains I could not follow these plans as a long term lifestyle change.

This year I became a Retired Dieter. This means I no longer will refuse to eat the foods I enjoy. I have stopped listening to the media talk about the latest new diet and fat loss craze. All diets have a hook, but at the end of the day it comes down to one thing, one way or another we have to eat less. So what is the solution?

For me the effective way to lose body fat, and control my weight , is by using intermittent fasting. Intermittent Fasting is simply taking times of fast (no food) and working them into your lifestyle. You still eat every day, but you will incorporate a period of up to 24hrs without food into your day.

Using Intermittent Fasting once or twice a week reduces body fat, yet still allows you to enjoy the foods you enjoy. On the days you are not fasting, you eat normally. Following the Intermittent Fasting lifestyle I am still cutting carbs from my diet. I am actually cutting carbs for the equivalent of 2 full days per week.

We could debate the theory, but I like to work on results. In my first seven weeks of using Intermittent Fasting for weight loss, I have reduced my body fat by 12% and lost 24lbs. In my 14 years of trying different diet plans, I have never had results that compare to these. The other main point is, unlike my experience of low carb diets, I have not felt restricted with Intermittent Fasting, I have not had any cravings for specific foods like I did with Low Carb dieting because no foods are off limits.

Why do I feel that intermittent fasting is something I can use as long term after only seven weeks? The answer is because on any diet I have tried in the past, I would always have days where I felt I was restricted, so the diet became difficult, and that is on the diets that I managed to stick to for seven weeks!

The difference with Intermittent Fasting is, it isn't a diet, because no foods are off limits. Once you have completed once fast, you know from that day forward, you can incorporate it into your lifestyle, how you do that, and how often you do it, is up to you, that is the great thing about Intermittent Fasting, it adapts to your lifestyle, in the past when you went on a diet, how often did it dominate your life? This again is a prime example why diets fail.

So my suggestion is if you are looking to reduce your body fat, and think you should reduce your carbs, try Intermittent Fasting. Become a Retired Dieter, and let me know how you get on.

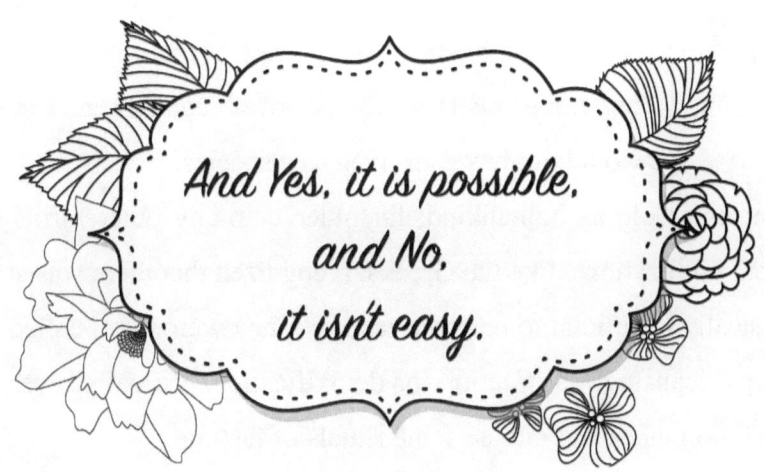

And Yes, it is possible, and No, it isn't easy.

CHAPTER 2
BRIEF HISTORY ON INTERMITTENT FASTING

Before the advent of agriculture, humans never ate three meals a day plus snacks in between. We ate only when we found food which could be hours or days apart. Hence, from an evolution standpoint, eating three meals a day is not a requirement for survival. Otherwise, we would not have survived as a species.

Fasting is as old as humankind, far older than any other forms of diets. Ancient civilizations, like the Greeks, recognized that there was something intrinsically beneficial to periodic fasting. They were often called times of healing, cleansing, purification, or detoxification. Virtually, every culture and religion on earth practice some rituals of fasting.

Today, experts tells us that lean people live longer and are more productive in their daily lives. For this reason, millions have embarked upon some sort of weight loss program. Although millions diet and exercise to live longer or feel better and have more energy, my guess is that the majority do so to look better. We aspire to the lean image portrayed by those we see on television, and print ads, and in movies.

Years ago, people who wanted to lose fat did so based upon a very limited amount of information — Before the invention of the word "calorie," people lost weight by fasting. Fasting was introduced to humankind by

God. The Jews fast, as do the Christians and Muslims. All do so because God told the prophets that abstaining from food was good for the soul as well as the physical body. A common physical change that all three groups noticed was a loss in weight, and a decrease in body fat. Thus, to lose weight, the first dieter would abstain from food and drink water. It was then, and is today, a proven way to lose fat, albeit an extreme approach.

When a person abstains from food, the body has to break down body tissue to use for survival. Most of this fuel comes from stored energy in the form of body fat reserves. Unfortunately, a severe fast is also a dangerous fast because the body also calls upon other tissues to be used as fuel. With fasting, the body chooses a mixture of stored body fat as fuel and lean body mass.

Lean body mass is readily tapped as fuel. Just as the body taps body fat and breaks it down to use as energy, it can do the same with muscle and organs. When deprived of food, the body can easily break down the heart, liver, and other organs to make fuel. The body will also rip apart the muscles throughout the body to make fuel during a starvation fast. While fat is burned up quickly as fuel, muscle and organs are also burned. This can lead to exhaustion and eventually death. So, we can conclude, the fast, while spiritually advantageous, isn't exactly the smartest approach to losing fat.

Once people figured out prolonged fasting works, but the negative outcome was death, they began to alter the fasting approach to weight loss.

Thus, the modified fast was born. Fast forward to the 21st century, we have all forgotten about this ancient practice.

After all, fasting is really bad for business! Food manufacturers encourage us to eat multiple meals and snacks a day. Nutritional authorities warn that skipping a single meal will have dire health consequences. Over time, these messages have been so well-drilled into our heads.

Intermittent fasting weight loss program is radically different from most weight loss programs being promoted in the market. However, its ideas are scientifically sound when it comes to losing weight. You should give this program a go if you are serious about weight loss.

Intermittent fasting has become quite the phenomenon these days. Recent studies showed that people who tried it have lost weight, increased health, and believed to have a long lifespan. Basically, intermittent fasting is a pattern of eating that alternates between period of fasting, usually consuming only water, and non-fasting, usually eating anything a person want no matter how fattening.In other words, a person can eat anything he wants during a 24-hour period and fast for the next 24 hours.

This approach to weight control seems to be supported by science, as well as religious and cultural practices around the globe. Adherents of intermittent fasting claim that this practice is a way to become more circumspect about food.The program is also recognized to prevent cognitive decline. Research was conducted in 2006 on mice, in which water maze tests were used to assess cognitive functions of mice on normal diet and those on intermittent fasting. It was discovered that mice put on intermittent fasting experienced slower cognitive declines, which too applies to human beings.

There are many different popular intermittent fasts and hundreds of more possible variations. There are two kinds of intermittent fasts that are most basic and frequently used. First, it's the daily fasting in which the person only gets to eat once every 20-28 hours within a 4-hour period. The second is fasting for 1-3x a week, also called alternate day fasting, in which a person eats anything he wants on one day and fast the whole of next day.

Intermittent fasting has many beneficial effects as tested on animals like rodents and primates. One study found that there has been a "reduced serum glucose and insulin levels and increased resistance of neurons in the brain to excitotoxic stress." In 2008, a study on intermittent fasting showed that lifespan increases of 40.4% and 56.6% in C. elegans for alternate day (24 hour) and two-of-each-three day (48 hour) fasting, respectively, as compared to an ad libitum diet. And a 2009 study showed that intermittent fasting on rats improved long-term survival after chronic heart failure via pro-angiogenic, anti-apoptotic and anti-remodeling effects. Researchers caution that only a few studies have been done on humans who are practicing intermittent fasts. The effects of exercise and meal frequency on body composition are an interesting but largely unexplored area of research.

However, there are some positive results. Just last month, the Proceedings of the National Academy of Sciences published a study showing that reducing calories 30% a day increased the memory function of the elderly. In 2007, the journal Free Radical Biology & Medicine published a study that showed asthma patients who fasted, had fewer symptoms, better airway function and a decrease in the markers of inflammation in the blood than those who didn't fast.

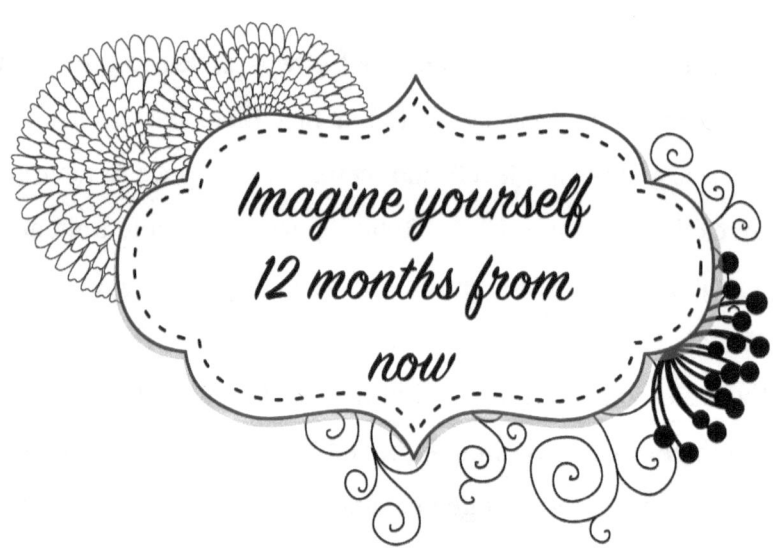

Imagine yourself 12 months from now

CHAPTER 3
BENEFITS OF INTERMITTENT FASTING

Everyone seems to be talking about intermittent fasting these days, including myself. The discussions range from the incredible to the incredulous about the benefits or lack thereof of skipping meals such as breakfast. I mean didn't they that breakfast is the healthiest and should be the most substantial meal of the day. This leads me to look at just three benefits of pursuing an intermittent fasting program.

Everyone always wonders what the next big secret in the dieting industry is... Specifically, people want to burn fat and build muscle while putting in as little effort as possible. They want it all, and sometimes that's asking a little too much. At-least with most programs.

The benefits of intermittent fasting are vast. Fasting gets a bad rap, but there is real science behind the technique of fasting, in particular, intermittent fasting. Many people think that someone who is fasting has an eating disorder, but nothing could be farther from the truth.

The truth is that in today's society, we eat far too much and too often. Our bodies are very precise mechanisms that, allowed to run properly, will take care of us far beyond our imagination. The problem lies with the fact that historically, for thousands and thousands of years, we were a species with little food resources and we worked long and hard each and every day for the morsels we did get. Today, we have a plethora of food, most of it very fattening, and sedentary lifestyles. This both contributes to obesity and disease.

Fasting intermittently can eliminate many problems that are caused by overeating and sitting around all day, instead of out hunting and gathering. The fact is that we have not evolved enough to be able to handle all the calories that we ingest on a daily basis, our bodies still operate as if we were hunter and gatherers. Not until the 20th century did most people have food at the ready, so 100 years is not even close to enough time to change how our body operates.

High blood pressure, high cholesterol, and obesity are all problems that can be helped with intermittent fasting. A particularly effective fasting plan is called the Fast 5. This plan requires you to fast for 19 hours everyday and eat for five consecutive hours. It is important to not that you DO eat when fasting intermittently. Eating is essential to your health, but eating once or twice a day during a short period is more natural to our bodies than stuffing them 12 out of 24 hours in a day. Again, up until the 20th century, most people only managed to eat once a day for thousands of years.

The pattern of eating called "Intermittent Fasting" usually means one fasts for a period of time and eats for a period of time. Many choose a 24 hour cycle of fasting, then eat healthy the next day, and continue this process as a lifestyle change.

Intermittent fasting can add 40%-56% more years to your life! That in itself is reason enough to do it. However other benefits include body weight reduction and fat oxidation.

When you fast your body is forced to scavenge for fuel thus removing aged and damaged cells in the process. This cleanses the body of undesirable and unwanted things and helps the weight loss and benefits of the good food choices be increased and more beneficial to your body.

Rats have been shown to have long-term and improved survival after heart failure after being on a IF eating plan, too. Researchers are also saying that it might help age related deficits in cognitive function, too, so that tells me that it might help ward off Alzheimer's Disease and other types of Dementia!

Your risk of heart disease and other heart ailments may also be decreased when you start a healthy intermittent fasting regimen. Your risk for other chronic illnesses and diseases will also most likely be reduced.

A healthier you can begin with intermittent fasting and healthy food choices! Keep carbs to 100 -150 grams per day. Many women eat between 1200-1500 calories per day, and when limiting their carbs, they are still losing weight. Men can handle up to 2000 calories per day. Of course, less is best, and you need to determine caloric intake based on your activity such as working hard and exercising.

Drink lots of fluids, especially water and exercise in the evenings if possible. This will help with those late night cravings.

Once you start eating and drinking healthier, your body won't crave as much (if any) junk food, so, making healthy food choices will get easier and easier as you progress in the intermittent fasting routine.

Alternate Day Fasting or ADF means alternating days of eating and not eating any food, but there is also an intermittent fasting called Modified Fasting where you consume about 20% of your normal calories one day and then eat normally (but healthy) the next day. This is often more attainable for people because they feel less deprived when they are able to at least eat something daily, and it still has most of the benefits of the ADF regimen.

But what if I told you there were programs ahead of the entire industry that could do that? Enter intermittent fasting.

A cell biologist Yoshinori Ohsumi has been able to develop a crucial process called Autography. After so many years of research and experiment he was awarded the Nobel Prize in Physiology or Medicine on Monday for discovering how cells recycle their content, a process known as autophagy, a Greek term for "self-eating."

But little was known about how autophagy happens, what genes were involved, or its role in disease and normal development until Dr. Ohsumi began studying the process in baker's yeast.

He later studies the process in other for cells to survive and to stay healthy. He discovered that autophagy genes and the metabolic pathways in yeast are used by higher organisms, including humans. And mutations in those genes can cause disease. His work led to a new field and inspired hundreds of researchers around the world to study the process and opened a new area of inquiry. He was the real founder of autophagy.

What is Autophagy?

Autophagy is a process by which cellular components are captured into organelles called autophagosomes and then brought to the lysosome or vacuole to be broke down and recycled for other use It frequently comes into play during starvation, allowing cells to survive periods of privation.

Research has been done on animals to find the benefits of this type of fasting, and you will be happy to know it can be beneficial to your health!

Here are the possible benefits of intermittent fasting

1. Improves Immune Function (Immune system booster)

The white blood cells of humans are an effective defense mechanism against pathogens in the body. However, white blood cells are limited by their ability to carry out their defensive function in entering cell and attacking intercellular pathogens. This is because the primary line of defense of these pathogens are in fact lysosomes. Lysosomes through a process known as autophagy, which means self-eating acts like the garbage disposal of the cell.

Damaged proteins, organelles, viruses, bacteria, and other pathogens are destroyed during autophagy. How long it is before your last meal directly impact lysosomal activities. Are you seeing the connection yet? The function of lysosomes is to control the amount of nutrients that are available to the cells for the organelles to use.

A filled stomach suppressed the functions of lysosomes and hence autophagy will not take place. Intermittent fasting allows the cells to undergo autophagy and hence lysosomes can carry out its garbage disposal function.

2. Better Health

You benefit from a better and improve health from the fact that a properly functioning immune system provides a more robust defence against pathogen in the body. The only way to remain healthy is to develop a strong and robust immune system in your body.

Choosing one of the feeding windows in intermittent fasting well help to regulate insulin response and glycemic loads in the body. You have heard many times that many lifestyle diseases are the result of too much sugar in the blood stream. That is the blood sugar level is too high. Diseases such as obesity and diabetes are all linked to this.

Intermittent Fasting or IF for short is not a diet or starvation process. It is an eating pattern. When one fasts and also reduce their calorie intake; it can lead to a healthier and prolonged life. Take note that our ancestors before us were gatherers and hunters. They did not have meals all the time and what they ate were based on what was available. With that being said, it means that our bodies are also designed to go for a few hours without eating. It can survive without having three square meals a day. Living the IF Life has many benefits which will be explained below.

Health Benefits

1. You keep yourself full. Some people think that fasting or dieting for that matter is equal to starvation. However, when Intermittent Fasting is done, Ghrelin which is a hormone that signals hunger adjusts to the new way of eating of the body which is why you will not feel hungry.

2. You will have better focus and improved concentration. When fasting, catecholamines, which is another hormone of the body is produced more. Therefore, the end result is that you will be more focused on what you are doing.

3. You will have more energy. Since you will not eat as much, there will be less wavering of blood sugar levels. This means that real energy will be more consistent. Plus, you lessen the risk of getting diabetes. You can also exercise while you are on fast which will actually boost your body's potential to burn more fats. A growth hormone is increased when you fast which help burn calories.

4. You burn more fat which means weight loss. Since you eat less and are taking in fewer calories, your body will turn into body fat to burn for energy instead of taking the energy from the food that is otherwise eaten on a regular basis if you are not on Intermittent Fasting. This also means that your body will show more of fits lean muscle mass. On a side note, if you are fasting for about 16 hours, your body is already consuming body fat.

5. You will also be able to benefit from the following:

- Less glucose in the blood and better insulin levels
- Less inflammation
- Protection against diseases such as heart disease, Alzheimer's, and cancers

A superb way to burn excess fat during a workout

The whole purpose of aerobic endurance training is to burn unwanted fat. Health conscious gym adherent are on a constant look out for ways to burn fat.As such a high-intensity exercise is one good way to cause the utilization of the body's fat storage instead of using glycogen.

You can increase fat utilization through ketosis by combining intermittent fasting and exercise. This is because your best fat burning work out is best done when your body is in a glycon depleted state.

Breakfast Is the most important meal of the day:

That myth is easily killed. Those who engage in regular fasting (often goes from sleep to lunch, meaning skipping breakfast) report increased focus, increased energy levels and better mood while fasting. Looking for your new coffee? You've found one that burns fat and gives you energy.

Eating Six Meals A Day Speeds Up The Metabolism:

If you are consuming the same number of calories and have the same macronutrient distribution (primarily talking about protein), consuming those calories and nutrients between six meals and one makes near 0 difference. Because at the end of the day with either method, there will be the same caloric deficit if I cut calories, and the same surplus if I add calories!

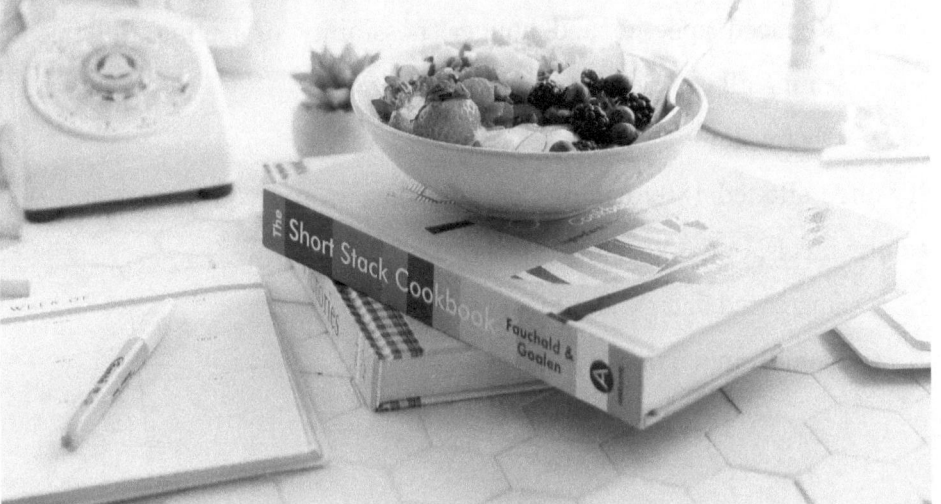

*With IF your
day is simpler
When you wake up,
you don't worry about
breakfast*

the fasting method.

By increasing insulin sensitivity, intermittent fasting can make sure when you are eating the calories are getting driven directly into your muscles! And when you aren't fasting the increased adrenaline/noradrenaline will give you energy and burn fat!

In the most simple sense, intermittent fasting is rotating between periods of eating, and periods of not eating. I'll list the benefits below, but the general reasoning behind participating in Intermittent fasting(IF) is that many people respond very well to eating most of their calories in less meals, especially while dieting.

This allows for hunger control, insulin sensitivity (read: muscle building) and more time for burning fat (increased adrenaline/noradrenaline).

Other Benefits of Intermittent fasting:

- Increased Insulin sensitivity/nutrient portioning, makes for a great way to build muscle without gaining fat!
- Increased adrenaline/noradrenaline, meaning more time spent burning fat!
- Reduced appetite and hunger, possibility of feeling full due to eating all calories in fewer meals
- **Example:**

If you're allotted 1800 calories on your diet, would you rather eat 2 900 calorie meals, or 6 300 calorie meals?

- Increased energy and focus
- And so much more...

This is everything you want in a diet. We want to reap all the benefits while building the body of our dreams and this is the perfect way to do it! This is how you accomplish the number one goal of the fitness industry... burning fat while building muscle!

Two Main Reasons Why You Should Do It:

1. Maximum Fat Loss:

The main reason why you should do it is that intermittent fasting consumes maximum fats. Just imagine, if you implement fasting just for two days a week, you are cutting a whole full two days calorie quota from your weekly consumption! And this combined with your daily workout can give excellent results and you will loss excessive fat.

2. Maintains workout load very well:

The second reason for fasting is that it allows you to maintain a moderate to intense workout load without losing your energy and metabolism. Most of the people think that fasting drains your energy and metabolism but that's not true. If you implement fasting in your diet plan, you will get more energy and a higher metabolism.

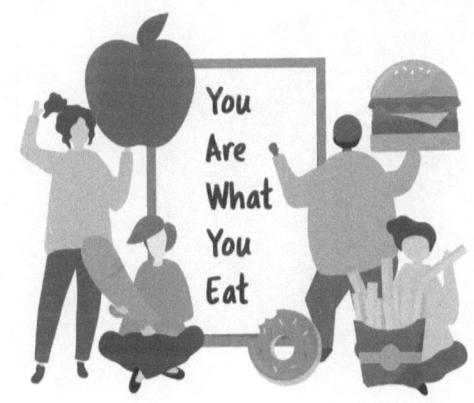

3. Its Beneficial Aspects:

The third reason why the fasting is a good practice to include in your workout plan is its beneficial aspects which give you great benefits. When you do any type of fasting, your body adjusts to it by consuming your body fat. It also has some psychological benefits, like you would feel that you are not a slave to food.

A little disclosure:

Intermittent fasting is way ahead of the rest of the industry. It goes against a lot of the mainstream myths that are currently being perpetuated and that you might believe. But then again, we have to ask ourselves, do we want mainstream results? Or do we want to be above average, unique and at the top? I know my answer.

CHAPTER 4
WHAT TO EXPECT

Intermittent fasting is a feeding pattern which alternates between periods of fasting and controlled eating. It is a simple dietary method divided into many types. One of the intermittent fasting methods is alternate day fasting, whereby a person takes a normal diet on particular days of the week and fasts on some. During the fasting days, one does not fully abstain from food but rather reduces calorie intake to 1/4 of the normal diet.

The other fasting type is whereby eating is restricted to a certain time window within a day. This means restricting eating between an eight hours window eating period, which means a person eats once in every eight hours. Some people however reduce the span to either six, four or even two hours according to their convenience. The longest time that a person can stay without food on intermittent fasting is 36 hours. If practiced accordingly, it can result in a number of positive health effects.

For instance, intermittent fasting promotes general good health. It significantly reduces cravings for snack foods and sugars. The practice normalizes insulin as well as leptin sensitivity. Insulin resistance contributes to many chronic diseases such as diabetes, cancer and heart infections. Intermittent fasting will therefore protect the body from such infections.

Intermittent fasting results in improved brain health. Fasting helps the body to convert stored glycogen into glucose to release energy. If the fasting proceeds for some time, continued breakdown of body fats induces the liver to secrete ketone bodies; these small molecules are by-products of fatty acids synthesis, and the brain can use them as fuel. Research also indicates that exercise and fasting results in genes and other growth factors which are essential in recycling and rejuvenating the brain.

This type of fasting also boosts body fitness and loss of weight. Combined fasting and exercise increases effects of catalysts and cellular factors so that breakdown of glycogen and fats is maximized. Exercising while hungry, therefore, forces the body to burn stored fats for significant weight loss.

Intermittent fasting will also boost muscle building especially in men. This is because after eating, the energy gained will be used to sustain a workout session. But if training is done while fasting, the body utilizes stored body fats to sustain the exercises. Eating after the session ensures that the energy gained is utilized in replenishing the body in the best way. This assists the muscles to quickly recover and build up.

In conclusion, intermittent fasting is a healthy practice but it could result in depression to people who cannot fully sustain it. It needs commitment and perseverance to move through the changes in diet, since only consistency will achieve these positive results.

Expect Weight Loss & Diabetes
Fasting has no standard duration. It may be done for a few hours to many

days to months on end. Intermittent fasting is an eating pattern where we cycle between fasting and regular eating. Shorter fasts of 16-20 hours are generally done more frequently, even daily. Longer fasts, typically 24-36 hours, are done 2-3 times per week. As it happens, we all fast daily for a period of 12 hours or so between dinner and breakfast.

Fasting has been done by millions for thousands of years. Is it unhealthy? No. In fact, numerous studies have shown that it has enormous health benefits.

What Happens When We Eat Constantly?

Before going into the benefits of intermittent fasting, it is best to understand why eating 5-6 meals a day or every few hours (the exact opposite of fasting) may do more harm than good. We ingest food energy whenever we eat. The key hormone involved is insulin (produced by the pancreas), which rises during meals. Both carbohydrates and protein stimulate insulin. Fat triggers a smaller insulin effect, but fat is rarely eaten alone.

Insulin has two major functions -

First, it allows the body to immediately start using food energy. Carbohydrates are rapidly converted into glucose, raising blood sugar levels. Insulin directs glucose into the body cells to be used as energy. Proteins are broken down into amino acids and excess amino acids may be turned into glucose. Protein does not necessarily raise blood glucose, but it can stimulate insulin. Fats have minimal effect on insulin.

49

Second, insulin stores away excess energy for future use. Insulin converts excess glucose into glycogen and store it in the liver. However, there is a limit to how much glycogen can be stored away. Once the limit is reached, the liver starts turning glucose into fat. The fat is then put away in the liver (in excess, it becomes fatty liver) or fat deposits in the body (often stored as visceral or belly fat).

Therefore, when we eat and snack throughout the day, we are constantly in a fed state and insulin levels remain high. In other words, we may be spending the majority of the day storing away food energy.

What Happens When We Fast?

The process of using and storing food energy that occurs when we eat goes in reverse when we fast. Insulin levels drop, prompting the body to start burning stored energy. Glycogen, the glucose that is stored in the liver, is first accessed and used. After that, the body starts to break down stored body fat for energy.

Thus, the body basically exists in two states - the fed state with high insulin and the fasting state with low insulin. We are either storing food energy or burning food energy. If eating and fasting are balanced, then there is no weight gain. There is a good chance that overtime we may end up gaining weight if we spend the majority of the day eating and storing energy.

Intermittent Fasting Versus Continuous Calorie-Restriction

The portion-control strategy of constant caloric reduction is the most common dietary recommendation for weight loss and type two diabetes.

For instance, the American Diabetes Association recommends a 500-750 kcal/day energy deficit coupled with regular physical activity. Dietitians follow this approach and recommend eating 4-6 small meals throughout the day.

Does the portion-control strategy work in the long-run? Rarely. A cohort study with a 9-year follow-up from the United Kingdom on 176,495 obese individuals indicated that only 3,528 of them succeeded in attaining normal body weight by the end of the study. That is a failure rate of 98%!

Intermittent fasting is not constant caloric restriction. Restricting calories causes a compensatory increase in hunger and worse, a decrease in the body's metabolic rate, a double curse! Because when we are burning fewer calories per day, it becomes increasingly harder to lose weight and much easier to gain weight back after we have lost it. This type of diet puts the body into a "starvation mode" as metabolism revs down to conserve energy.

Intermittent fasting does not have any of these drawbacks.

Unlike a daily caloric reduction diet, intermittent fasting raises metabolism. This makes sense from a survival standpoint. If we do not eat, the body uses stored energy as fuel so that we can stay alive to find another meal. Hormones allows the body to switch energy sources from food to body fat.

Studies demonstrate this phenomenon clearly. For instance, four days of continuous fasting increased Basal Metabolic Rate by 12%. Levels of the neurotransmitter norepinephrine, which prepares the body for action, increased by 117%. Fatty acids in the bloodstream increased over 370% as the body switched from burning food to burning stored fats.

No loss in muscle mass

Unlike a regular calorie-restriction diet, intermittent fasting does not burn muscles as many have feared. In 2010, researchers looked at a group of subjects who underwent 70 days of alternate daily fasting (ate one day and fasted the next). Their muscle mass started off at 52.0 kg and ended at 51.9 kg. In other words, there was no loss of muscles, but they did lose 11.4% of fat and saw major improvements in LDL cholesterol and triglyceride levels.

During fasting, the body naturally produces more human growth hormone to preserve lean muscles and bones. Muscle mass is generally preserved until body fat drops below 4%. Therefore, most people are not at risk of muscle-wasting when doing intermittent fasting.

Reverses insulin resistance, type 2 diabetes, and fatty liver

Type-2 diabetes is a condition whereby there is simply too much sugar in the body, to the point that the cells can no longer respond to insulin and take in any more glucose from the blood (insulin resistance), resulting in high blood sugar. Also, the liver becomes loaded with fat as it tries to clear out the excess glucose by converting it to and storing it as fat. Therefore, to reverse this condition, two things have to happen - First, stop putting more sugar into the body. Second, burn the remaining sugar off.

The best diet to achieve this is a low-carbohydrate, moderate-protein, and high-healthy fat diet, also called ketogentic diet. (Remember that carbohydrate raises blood sugar the most, protein to some degree, and fat the least.) That is why a low-carb diet will help reduce the burden of incoming glucose. For some people, this is already enough to reverse insulin resistance and type-2 diabetes. However, in more severe cases, diet alone is not sufficient.

What about exercise? Exercise will help burn off glucose in the skeletal muscles but not all the tissues and organs, including the fatty liver. Clearly, exercise is important, but to eliminate the excess glucose in the organs, there is the need to temporarily "starve" the cells.

Intermittent fasting can accomplish this. That is why historically, people called fasting a cleanse or a detox. It can be a very powerful tool to get rid of all the excesses. It is the fastest way to lower blood glucose and insulin levels, and eventually reversing insulin resistance, type-2 diabetes, and fatty liver.

By the way, taking insulin for type-2 diabetes does not address the root cause of the problem, which is excess sugar in the body. It is true that insulin will drive the glucose away from the blood, resulting in lower blood glucose, but where does the sugar go? The liver is just going to turn it all into fat, fat in the liver and fat in the abdomen. Patients who go on insulin often end up gaining more weight, which worsens their diabetes.

Enhances heart health

Over time, high blood glucose from type-2 diabetes can damage the blood vessels and nerves that control the heart. The longer one has diabetes, the higher the chances that heart disease will develop. By lowering blood sugar through intermittent fasting, the risk of cardiovascular disease and stroke is also reduced.

Also, intermittent fasting has been shown to improve blood pressure, total and LDL (bad) cholesterol, blood triglycerides, and inflammatory markers associated with many chronic diseases.

Boosts brain power

Multiple studies showed that fasting has many neurologic benefits including attention and focus, reaction time, immediate memory, cognition, and generation of new brain cells. Mice studies also showed that intermittent fasting reduces brain inflammation and prevents the symptoms of Alzheimer's.

What To Expect With Intermittent Fasting

Hunger Goes Down

We normally feel hunger pangs about four hours after a meal. So, if we fast for 24 hours, does it mean that our hunger sensations will be six times more severe? Of course not.

Many people are concerned that fasting will result in extreme hunger and overeating. Studies showed that on the day after a one-day fast, there is, indeed, a 20% increase in caloric intake. However, with repeated fasting, hunger and appetite surprisingly decrease.

Hunger comes in waves. If we do nothing, the hunger dissipates after a while. Drinking tea (all kinds) or coffee (with or without caffeine) is often enough to fight it off. However, it is best to drink it black. Do not use any types of sugar or artificial sweeteners. bone broth can also be taken during fasting if necessary.

Blood sugar does not crash

Sometimes people worry that blood sugar will fall very low during fasting and they will become shaky and sweaty. This does not happen as blood sugar is tightly monitored by the body and there are multiple mechanisms to keep it in the proper range. During fasting, the body begins to break down glycogen in the liver to release glucose. This happens every night during our sleep.

If we fast for longer than 24-36 hours, glycogen stores become depleted and the liver will manufacture new glucose using glycerol which is a by-product of the breakdown of fat (a process called gluconeogenesis). Apart from using glucose, our brain cells can also use

ketones for energy. Ketones are produced when fat is metabolized and they can supply up to 75% of the brain's energy requirements (the other 25% from glucose).

The only exception is for those who are taking diabetic medications and insulin. You MUST first consult your doctor as the dosages will probably need to be reduced while you are fasting. Otherwise, if you overmedicate and hypoglycemia develops, which can be dangerous, you must have some sugar to reverse it. This will break the fast and make it counterproductive.

The dawn phenomenon

After a period of fasting, especially in the morning, some people experience high blood glucose. This dawn phenomenon is a result of the circadian rhythm whereby just before awakening, the body secretes higher levels of several hormones to prepare for the upcoming day -

Adrenaline - to give the body some energy

Growth hormone - to help repair and make new protein

Glucagon - to move glucose from storage in the liver to the blood for use as energy

Cortisol, the stress hormone - to activate the body

These hormones peak in the morning hours, then fall to lower levels during the day. In non-diabetics, the magnitude of the blood sugar rise is small and most people will not even notice it. However, for the majority of the diabetics, there can be a noticeable spike in blood glucose as the liver dumps sugar into the blood.

This will happen in extended fasts too. When there is no food, insulin levels stay low while the liver releases some of its stored sugar and fat. This is natural and not a bad thing at all. The magnitude of the spike will decrease as the liver becomes less bloated with sugar and fat.

Who Should Not Do Intermittent Fasting?

- Women who want to get pregnant, are pregnant, or breastfeeding.
- Those who are malnourished or underweight.
- Children under 18 years of age and elders.
- Those who have gout.
- Those who have a gastroesophageal reflux disease (GERD).
- Those who have eating disorders should first consult with their doctors. Those who are taking diabetic medications and insulin must first consult with their doctors as dosages will need to be reduced.

- Those who are taking medications should first consult with their doctors as the timing of medications may be affected.
- Those who feel very stressed or have cortisol issues should not fast because fasting is another stressor.
- Those who are training very hard most days of the week should not fast.

How To Prepare For Intermittent Fasting?

If anyone is thinking about starting intermittent fasting, it is best to first switch to a low-carbohydrate, high-healthy fat diet for three weeks. This will allow the body to become accustomed to using fat rather than glucose as a source of energy. That means getting rid of all sugars, grains (bread, cookies, pastries, pasta, rice), legumes, and refined vegetable oils. This will minimize most side effects associated with fasting.

Start with a shorter fast of 16 hours, for instance, from dinner (8 pm) until lunch (12 pm) the next day. You can eat normally between 12 pm and 8 pm, and you can eat either two or three meals. You can extend the fast to 18, 20 hours once you feel comfortable with it.

For shorter fasts, you can do it every day, continuously. For more extended fasts, such as 24-36 hours, you can do it 1-3 times a week, alternating between fasting and normal eating days.

There is no single fasting regimen that is correct. The key is to choose one that works best for you. Some people achieve results with shorter fasts, others may need longer fasts. Some people do a classic water-only fast, others do a tea and coffee fast. No matter what you do, it is essential to stay hydrated and monitor yourself. If you feel ill at any point, you should stop immediately. You can be hungry, but you should not feel sick.

You are 10-13 hours into your first fast and trying to wait 2 and a half more hours before eating. All you can think about is food...

SOLUTIONS:

- You can drink plain green or black tea to help push through the hunger.

- Drink some hot water with a twist of pink Himalayan salt in it and stay busy.

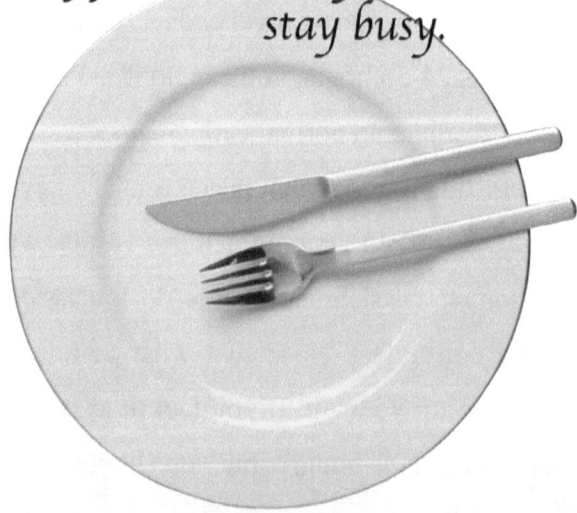

CHAPTER 5
HOW TO START INTERMITTENT FASTING

Intermittent fasting can improve health, reduce the risk of serious illness, and promote longevity. Perhaps you're intrigued and would like to give it a go, but aren't sure how to start. Or maybe you have tried it once or twice and found it too challenging. I will give you strategies and guidelines to practice intermittent fasting safely and successfully.

Intermittent fasting is without a doubt one of the fastest and most efficient ways to lose body-fat and do better. Daily fasting is becoming the lifestyle of choice for many people looking for health and fat loss benefits without complication. Here, are a few steps to starting out on a daily fasting lifestyle.

So what is daily fasting? While many people use the eating pattern in different ways; a basic definition might be a regular period of under-eating or no eating followed by a short "eating window." The first question many people have is "why do this?". Without going into the science (which is both well-documented and pretty compelling), it is easy to see why a daily fast is a good thing. Having many hours every day without eating is clearly going to lead to fat-loss, and the link between fat-loss and health should be obvious.

So what time period should you choose for daily fasting? Although there are many different possibilities depending on goals, lifestyle and situation, a common plan might be a 16 hour fast followed by 8 hours of eating. While this might seem like a long time to go without food, it is worth thinking about what this really means. Most people fast for at least ten hours overnight. A 16 hour fast is simply stretching this until lunchtime.

The beauty of this style of eating is threefold.

Firstly, it actually makes organizing your life easier. Rather than having to find a particular food choice at a particular time, you are simply not eating!

Secondly, a fasting lifestyle is less restrictive than other possibilities. This does not mean that you can eat doughnuts for eight hours, but it is not necessary to stick to celery either. Once you have taken in some protein (meat, fish, eggs) and fruit or vegetables (which should be the basis of any meal plan), you can certainly eat some of your favourite food. In eight hours after filling up on good food already, it is difficult to over-eat on rubbish.

Thirdly, and perhaps most importantly, this can become a lifestyle. Dropout rates for most diets are well over 90% after a week or to simply because it demands a lot of willpower to be hungry all the time and not eat until you aren't hungry. Here you can actually fill up during your eating window and many people (myself included) report feeling more alert during the fast.

How to Start

Seeking the help of a professional is advisable before you start fasting. However, you can start by choosing a day to skip breakfast. You can choose to have water or tea in lieu of breakfast. As you progress, try to go further by skipping lunch. You can take a normal sized meal if you feel that you need to eat or are feeling anxious.

When you start don't make your fast too long or too short

An ideal fast length for weight-loss and health benefits is between 16 and 24 hours depending on age, experience, and exact goals. Any less than this won't really give you the results you want (remember you are already fasting for 10-12 hours overnight) and any longer than this is simply unnecessary and can be harder to adapt to.

Increase your water intake when fasting

Intermittent fasting will also help to cleanse your system and let your body work more efficiently. You should increase your water intake to help this process. The best way to do this is have a glass/bottle of water with you at all times so that you can sip regularly.

Break your fast with a healthy meal

The first thing you eat after a fast should be a healthy meal. Apart from the obvious benefits of eating healthy food, this also leaves less space for eating junk. Given that you might only have eight hours to eat your daily food, filling up on the good stuff first is always a good option.

Time your food around your workouts

It goers without saying that working out should be part of any healthy eating plan. The centre piece of your training efforts should be weight-training or bodyweight training. Try to eat most of your food in the period immediately after your workout. In this way, your body will be more likely to use these calories to rebuild and repair rather than be stored as fat.

Don't sweat the details

One of the real benefits of intermittent fasting is that it is not necessary to count calories or grams of macronutrients. This can be a pain and makes diets difficult to stick to. Follow principles and the details will take care of themselves.

Contra-Indications: Avoid intermittent fasting if you are pregnant, diabetic, suffering from a serious illness, or taking any prescribed medications. If in doubt, it is best to consult with your health care provider.

How To Start Losing Weight Simply By Intermittent Fasting

Now, I know you might be thinking: fasting? Is this going to be good? What are the benefits and how does it work?

All I ask is that you sit back, relax and enjoy what you are going to read: Keep and open mind. Intermittent fasting is a plan based on a 16-8 fasting to feeding window. What this means is that you fast for 16 hours and feed for eight hours. Simple, right? This is entirely based on your lifestyle. It does not necessarily mean that you should fast for straight for 16 hours.

Remember this is a lifestyle diet. It has to fit with your schedule. Make sure you structure your feeding and fasting around times that are very comfortable for you. If for some reason you can fast for 16 hours, don't stress it. It is OK to occasionally end your eating window early, especially if it passes the eight hour mark.

So how do you start?

Before you change your nutrition, I want to point out that for most people, this can be a great cause of stress. It is going to take gradual steps. Do not think that it will be easy, it wont. But with the right attitude and plan, you will see positive changes. Also, discard the "Oh no, I do not get to eat till 2 pm today! This is going to be hard" attitude. It will not help you. Instead, think of it as a gradual process which you incorporate and take it one day at a time. With that being said, you can start with the 12/12 split.

What does the 12/12 split mean? The 12/12 split means that you fast for 12 hours and then eat for the next 12 hours. Meaning that you can start fasting from 7 am to 7 pm and eating from 7 pm to 7 am. The one good thing about this is that you do not need to make drastic adjustments to your feeding schedule. You might have to put off breakfast or shift dinner a bit, but that is all. Very easy and quick to implement. When you start experimenting with the 12/12 split, you might find out that you are snacking in the evening. Or that you might wake up in the middle of the night just to stuff things down your throat. This is a case of eating out of habit as opposed to being actually hungry.

7 pm - 7 am   **7 am - 7 pm**

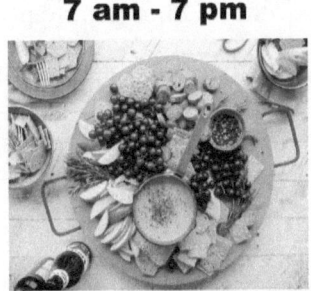

Tips and advice to help you get started immediately

- First, intermittent fasting isn't a diet. It's simply a schedule for eating.
- Start small and give yourself attainable goals. Make sure you know what you are getting into; it is all a thing of the mind, so mental preparation is key. Start small and evaluate your performance as you go. *Example*: start with just 2 days a week. If it is easy - start with 5 days the next week (every work day), skipping breakfast and having breakfast and lunch on weekends.
- Try signing up for an online program to help you calculate and monitor your calories from your current plan and help you switch over to fewer meals per day (which supports intermittent fasting).
- Remember that it is a lifestyle change, so it should be structured around your lifestyle. Do what makes you comfortable.
- Put a picture somewhere you could see of when you were thinner.
- Try to fall in love with water.
- Stay off the scale for 1 month at a time.
- Move your eating window around each day if you want the flexibility. Other people prefer a set eating window.
- Follow the fast you have outlined for that week.
- Start going to the gym 3x a week.
- The first week is the most difficult. After a few weeks, you really do train yourself to eat during the window and not always feel hungry.

In many cases, people 'give up' intermittent fasting because they simply tried to change too much too soon.

They dove into fasting, changed their diet, began an exercise program and forfeited getting a little sloshed on the weekend. It's just too much all at once.

The best way you'll know is to try. This is 99% experimental. You'll discover what works best for you, for your body, your social plans, your work, your family.

Can I start my fasting 7 pm evening till 1 pm afternoon?

- There is no right or wrong in fasting. Fast when it works best for you.

Are there any foods off limits?

- I just recommend 85-90% if your daily foods are from whole, natural sources and the other 10-15% can be from sources outside of that. It's all about calorie intake vs calorie output though. If your goal is to lose weight, you still have to watch the amount of those foods that you're eating and burning more calories a day than you eat!

- I really depends on your goals. Some do keto, some eat whatever they want within their food windows.

Is doing 12-13 hours of fasting is okay for weight loss?

- When you are just starting it's good to make a little break. But if you will lose weight I recommend 16 hours.

How Can I Lose A Stone In A Month

Rapid, Yet Sustained Weight Loss. One month, one stone, one concerted effort. Lets figure out what's necessary to achieve this. If we assume 30 days for a month, then we need to lose about 5lbs every ten days (about 2kg, or 15lb in 30 days, or 0.5lb/day, or over 3lbs per week).

I'm going to take an imaginary man and woman and put some figures down for them, showing you how to do it for yourself if you're different from my examples.

If we assume that there are about 3500 calories in a pound of fat, then you need to create a deficit of at least 11500 calories each week if you want to get those 3lbs off (3500 x 14lbs = 49000cals).

If we then break that down into each day, that's a daily deficit of about 1600 calories. Now, let's find out how much energy it costs to stay living: I'll take 3 men and 3 women.

Male 1
70kg -11st 0.3lb - 154.3lbs
Energy cals (range) 1,918 - 3,036

Male 2
80kg - 12st 8.4lb - 176.4lbs
Energy cals (range) 2,038 - 3,226

Male 3
90kg - 14st 2.4lb - 198.4lbs
Energy cals (range) 2,158 - 3,416

Female 1
60kg - 9st 6.3lb - 132.3lbs

Energy cals (range) 1,598 - 2,531

Female 2
70kg -11st 0.3lb - 154.3lbs
Energy cals (range) - 1,718 - 2,721

Female 3
80kg - 12st 8.4lb - 176.4lbs
Energy cals (range) - 1,838 - 2,911

Notes: The ranges shown for daily calorie expenditure are dependent on activity level, from sedentary (think office worker that drives to work and takes no or very limited exercise) to highly active (someone who has an job that involves several hours of manual labour per day, or exercises for more than 90 mins at a high intensity/consistently high heart rate each day).

These imaginary figures are based upon someone being about 170 cm tall, in their mid 30's, and are used for illustration purposes only, the principles behind the practices here are valid, you need to personalize the practices to your situation. These are estimations only and will vary person to person, to find out more accurately you need to get your own starting figures. You can do this using the calculators found at caloriesperhour.com. Use the BMR and RMR calcs for a rough starting point, then use the practices here to modify the figures based on real world results.

So you can see that for a woman of 60 kg, who is only lightly active or sedentary, this would basically mean not eating at all, for about a month!

Who is this for? Thing is though, a 60 kg woman doesn't really need to lose 14lbs (about 6kg) or over 10% of her bodyweight, so we're not catering for this person. What we should be looking at is the higher end of the scale. That's where big weight loss numbers are really practical.

If, for example you look at the 90 kg man, even a sedentary individual could cut over 1000 cals from their daily intake, as long as they do it with the right foods. I'll come on to that in a moment.

First, let's take a brief look at the three factors that will make this massive calorie reduction possible.

Intermittent Fasting

Eating high protein, low fat, low carb.

Doing only high-intensity weights and very low intensity cardio.

Now let's expand each of those so you can create your own plan.

1: Intermittent Fasting

Intermittent Fasting (the Leangains version) is a simple approach to feeding the body. You split the day into two phases, an eating phase, and a non-eating phase. The eating phase lasts around eight hours, therefore the fasting phase lasts about 16 hours. This doesn't mean that you eat for the whole of the 8-hour block!

There are two key aspects to IF that make it work in your favour when it comes to massive weight loss.

1: Each day is split, physiologically, into two distinct phases, each of which help your fat loss goal. These two phases are an anabolic, or tissue building phase, and a fat burning, or energy breakdown phase.

2: Eating High Protein, Low Fat, Low Carb

In his superb set of articles about designing a fat loss diet, Lyle MacDonald talks about setting things up from the ground, rather than the top. Say what? Well, what we've done here starts with a weight loss goal, that being the top or end point, and the worked backward to figure out what we need to do. In those articles Lyle takes a slightly different approach and figures out what you need physiologically, and then puts those figures into a diet, to see what comes out at the end.

Here, we are going to use part of that approach (setting protein intake) to give you a starting point for figuring out your foods.

How much food do you need?

Or more specifically, how much protein should you be aiming for at each meal? Well, we can give two answers to that question, the answer that's best is the one that makes you feel most reassured. The quick answer is 'lots'. The more specific answer is worked out as follows; start with a level of about 1g/lb of bodyweight and divide over your two or three meals, and then adjust based on lean tissue and strength drops and hunger/satiety levels. So, if you find your strength dropping, and your muscle leaving your body, you need to add more protein in, and if you find yourself getting hungry between meals or not satisfied at a meal, add more protein!

Why start with a statement like that?

Because, it's too easy for many people to drop back into old ways of 'exercising for weight loss.'

What you NEED to be doing is heavy weights, with low reps and using as big movements as possible. Remember, big weights are specific to each individual, and the actual number/weight is irrelevant, what's important is that you lift to YOUR capacity and you learn how to fully lift at your capacity. For those of you that have hardly lifted weights before that means learning what a maximum effort lift feels like, AND expecting that max to go up quickly as you learn how to get more and more out of yourself.

The great thing about this program is that it really is simple. Take the following exercises and rotate them:

Squat

- Dumbell press, bench press or bodyweight dips
- Dumbell or barbell shoulder press
- Lat pulldown, pullup, seated row or bent over barbell/dumbell row
- Deadlift.

Your rotation is simple: Do 3 weeks of 5 set sof 4-6 reps (5x5 style routine) and then three weeks of three sets of 9-12 reps (3x10 style routine). Each time you hit the upper rep range you increase the weight. Only after 10-14 weeks do you need to rest (but if you've already been exercising consistently for more than 12 weeks, you need to take a week of total rest right now - unless you're goal is within 12 weeks from the start of your program, in which case, you get your rest at the end of that!) If you don't know how to do these exercises, you can get instruction from a competent trainer (you can find if they're any good by watching how they get you to move and focus on the exercises your learning, if they get you to do your exercises like those done in instruction videos you may be sure they know their stuff), or you can check out the copious amount of vids on YouTube and figure your way.

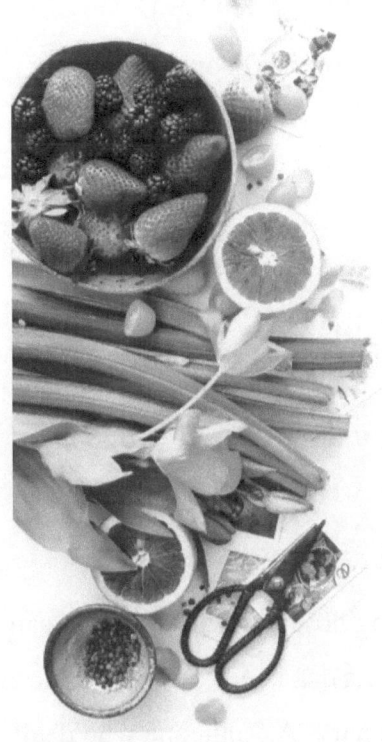

Anytime that you are not eating, you are fasting

CHAPTER 6
HOW LONG SHOULD I FAST

Eat Stop Eat - Flexible Intermittent Fasting Program

One of the most interesting weight loss methods I've encountered recently revolves around flexible intermittent fasting. It was created by Brad Pilon. The entire system which

Brad, a nutritionist and experienced trainer, has developed is called Eat Stop Eat. The supposition at its foundation is that you can eat relatively freely on most days of the week as long as you fast on one or two of them, and incorporate physical activity, mostly weight training, into your routine.

After I read the Eat Stop Eat manual (amazing how much information can be entered into something just 78 pages long), I knew that this was a method which was on the border of revolutionary. As someone who deals with diet and fitness issues, and educates people, I teach that fasting is usually bad for you. In fact, it can be beneficial as a cleansing process every few months, but if used too often, it can slow your metabolism down.

Here was Brad Pilon, in his Eat Stop Eat book, preaching to fast regularly as a way of life. I actually corresponded with Brad a few times just to make sure I got his system down right.

First of all, you should know that Brad is a respected nutritionist and researcher. His belief in flexible, intermittent fasting is based on research that he himself conducted, so it's not some unfounded theory.

Second, what Brad discovered was that our metabolism doesn't slow down that much if we limit our fasting period to 24 hours or so. What this fasting does help our body do is cleanse itself, and it creates an immediate calorie deficit (which is necessary for any weight loss). Putting these 2 together helps us lose weight faster and also improves our health.

- On training days, eat 9 hours of the day and fast the remaining 15.
- On off or cardio days, eat 6 hours of the day and fast the remaining 18.
- Weight training 3 days per week
- Cardio 2-4 times per week
- Eat maintenance + 500 calories on weight training days
- Eat 50% of maintenance on other days
- Majority of carbohydrate intake is on weight training days

Again, this plan is specific to fat loss. Plans for mass gain (bulking) and maintenance will be coming soon. Now for the detailed explanation of:

How to set up an Intermittent Fasting Diet for Fat Loss
- **Establishing Eating / Fasting Times**

The time of day in which you eat depends on if you are lifting weights that day, or not. On lifting days, your eating window is nine hours and on off or cardio days, its six hours. You will need to be able to weight train and do cardio at the same time of day, as this will throw off the schedule.

Eating schedule for weight training days

The fast is broken by a pre-workout shake, 15-30 minutes before you being your workout and lasts for nine hours. For instance, since I workout at 1pm, my eating window begins at 12:30 pm and lasts until 9:30 pm. This can be inconvenient if you workout at say, 8 pm, so I feel weightlifting at lunchtime or in the morning works best.

Next, we will look at setting up a schedule for off days or cardio days.

- **Eating schedule for off or cardio days**

The fast is broken an hour after cardio is complete and lasts for 6 hours. In my case, I do cardio at 1pm, so my fast is broken at 3pm. It remains 3pm on off days.

Summary

Monday: Fast ends at 12:30pm and begins at 9:30pm

Tuesday: Fast ends at 3:00pm and begins at 9:00pm

Wednesday: Fast ends at 12:30pm and begins at 9:30pm

Thursday: Fast ends at 3:00pm and begins at 9:00pm

Friday: Fast ends at 12:30pm and begins at 9:30pm

Saturday: Fast ends at 3:00pm and begins at 9:00pm

Sunday: Fast ends at 3:00pm and begins at 9:00pm

CHAPTER 7
WHAT TO CONSUME

You can eat wat you want and don't count the calories. Whilst fasting you can and should drink :

- plenty of water to avoid dehydration,
- tea and black coffee,
- unflavored mineral water,
- unflavored sparkling water
- unflafored seltzer.

Here are some tips and advice on how to drink more water during Intermittent Fasting:

- Try different sparkling waters
- Drink better water
- In the morning right after waking up, drink one glass of water
- Set little goals for yourself each day.
- Add small cuts of cucumber, lemon, strawberries, lemon grass, mint & sage or Himalayan salt in a small amount.
- Keep it accessible as possible. Have all kinds of cups with ice water just randomly around.
- Try water when it's at room temperature or when it is iced.

Coffee

Is coffee the key to weight loss while fasting?? The key is probably pushing it... But it definitely does help, and black coffee doesn't break your fast, so let's dive in!

Here are some questions about coffee:

What effects does a splash of creamer have in my coffee?
- Cream would break your fast. Get used to drinking more icy water; it is so refreshing... especially in the warmer months.

- You can save the coffee with creamer for your eating window!

You are trying to drink it, but you just can't stand black coffee. You absolutely cannot drink it plain. You just can't. What can you do?

- Never say "I can't." Yes, you can. You just have to decide to not have coffee in the morning.

- Try caffeine pills or tea.

- Start your fast after your coffee.

- You can try to switch to tea.

- Buy the Starbucks Cold Brew Medium Roast in the fridge section at a grocery store. Drink it over ice. It's good. Be sure to buy the unsweetened one.

- Try cold brew coffee or instant espresso.

- Try some different brands: Maxwell House, Folgers, Lavazza, Cafe Bustelo, Nescafe, Blond Roast, Darker Roasts, Dunkin Dark Roast, "Nitro" coffee at Starbucks, The San Francisco brand from Costco, Kirkland, Kuerig Starbucks blonde roast.

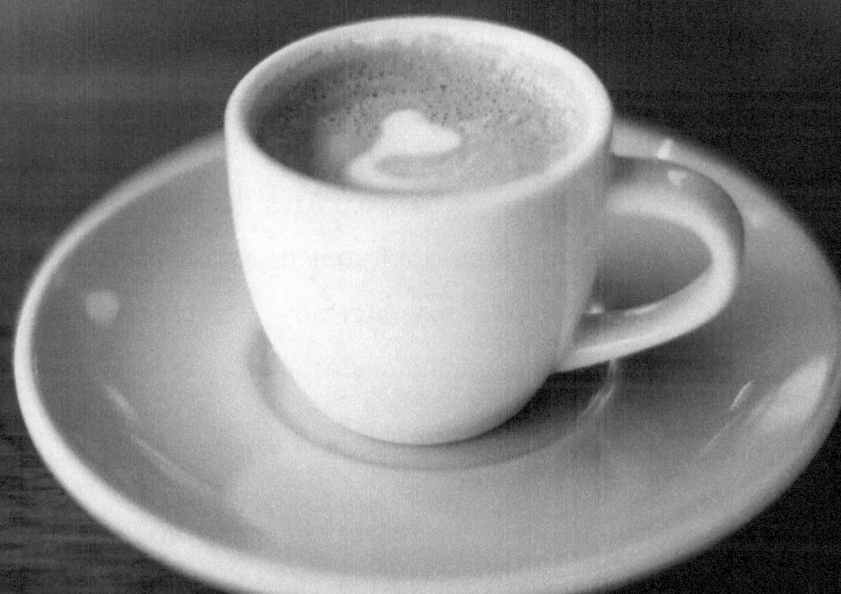

- Can I drink coffee with milk during IF?

- Milk/cream would break your fast.

Adding milk/cream/sugar will break your fast due to a consumption of calories.

- A French press brings out a lot of flavor, and the lighter the coffee, the more caffeine. As you roast the bean, the caffeine burns out.

- Try it iced instead.

Tea

Tea – black, white, green. Any of it is okay. No sweeteners. But can I have some herbal chamomile to sleep?

- Yes, you can do herbal teas. Just don't do herbal teas with fruit additives, like peach or raspberry.

Whatever your diet is whether its healthy or not you should see weight loss after about 3 weeks of intermittent fasting and do not be discouraged if you don't notice much progress at first, it's not a race and its better to lose weight in a linear fashion over time rather than crash losing a few pounds which you will put straight back on. After the first month you may want to take a look at your diet on non fasting days and cut out high sugar foods and any junk that you may normally eat. I have found that intermittent fasting over the long term tends to make me want to eat more healthy foods as a natural course.

Breakfast is the most important meal of the day:

That myth is easily killed. Those who engage in regular fasting (often goes from sleep to lunch, meaning skipping breakfast) report increased focus, increased energy levels and better mood while fasting. Looking for your new coffee? You've found one that burns fat and gives you energy.

Eating 6 Meals A Day Speeds Up The Metabolism:

If you are consuming the same number of calories and have the same macronutrient distribution (primarily talking about protein), consuming those calories and nutrients between six meals and one makes almost zero difference. Because at the end of the day with either method, there will be the same caloric deficit if I cut calories, and the same surplus if I add calories! And if there was a difference; I am inclined to believe that it is in favor of the fasting method.

By increasing insulin sensitivity, intermittent fasting can make sure when you are eating the calories are getting driven directly into your muscles! And when you aren't fasting the increased adrenaline/noradrenaline will give you energy and burn fat!

In the most simple sense, intermittent fasting is rotating between periods of eating and periods of not eating. I'll list the benefits below, but the general reasoning behind participating in Intermittent fasting (IF) is that many people respond very well to eating most of their calories in less meals, especially while dieting.

This allows for hunger control, insulin sensitivity (read: muscle building) and more time for burning fat (increased adrenaline/noradrenaline).

Macronutrient breakdown for weight training days:

Fat:

It doesn't matter where the fat comes from, as long as ten of these grams are in the form of Omega-3 Fish Oil.

Protein:

To determine the minimum amount of protein per day, you multiply your weight by 1.25. Our 200 lb person will need a minimum of 25 g of protein to preserve muscle. Sources don't really matter, just be sure to be mindful that you don't exceed the fat limit. Chicken, very lean red meat, fat free cheese and protein powder (whey or casein) are excellent choices.

Carbohydrates:

Carbohydrates makes up the remaining calories in your diet. Once again, sources don't matter, just be sure not to exceed the 30 g fat limit and be you want to keep sugar below 100 grams.

Try to get two large servings of veggies into your window everyday. You can close your eating window with a smoothie: like milk, vanilla protein powder, blueberries, banana, strawberries and spinach.

Diet for Off or Cardio Days

The eating window is shorter since calories are greatly reduced on off or cardio days. It works best to have 2-3 good size meals, rather than the 6-7 you read about in muscle mags.

On cardio days, the fast is broken with a 50 g protein shake, one hour after cardio is complete. Two hours after the shake, have your first "real" meal and continue until the six hours are up. As I mentioned earlier, carbs are limited to 20 per day and should consist of fibrous green vegetables and the trace amounts in food.

What to eat during the 8 hour window?

- You can eat what you want, but make sure you are eating enough during the 8 hours. You don't want your body to think it is in starvation mode, which makes losing weight harder.

What to eat and not gain weight?

- You just try to eat fairly healthy 80% of the time. Not processed food. What is processed food? Processed food is food not in its natural state. Anything pre-packaged or boxed is generally considered processed. The more ingredients that you can't pronounce, the more processed it is. Processed occurs along a spectrum. An apple is not processed. It is in its natural state. Freeze dried apples have been processed.

- When you fast for an extended period (16-18 hours), your body will crave foods that are better for you. Your body deserves quality - don't settle for less! Also, make sure you are getting plenty of healthy fats (nuts, avocado, salmon). You'll feel satisfied and less likely to overeat refined carbs.

- You can eat whatever you want, but you no longer want to eat whatever you want. Your wants and tastes will be changed so much after some months of IF.

- If you are trying this for the first time, it is your opportunity to get out of the diet mentality. Don't focus so much on weight loss at first, just freedom. Learn to pick and choose what works for you along the way.

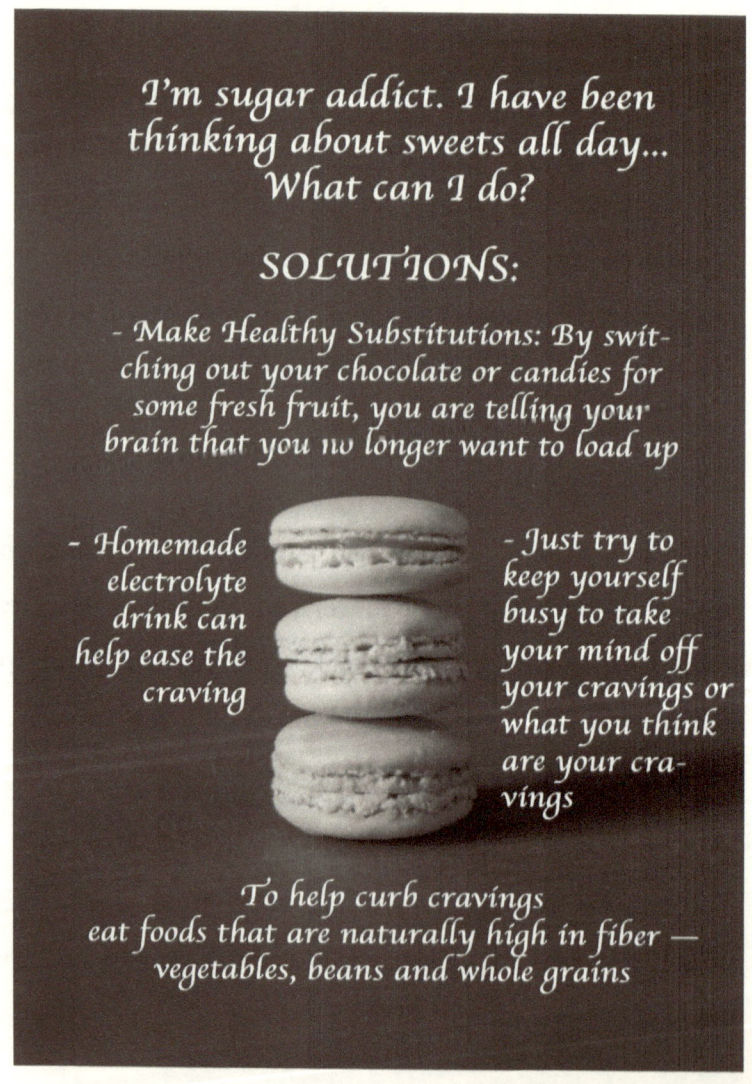

I'm sugar addict. I have been thinking about sweets all day... What can I do?

SOLUTIONS:

- Make Healthy Substitutions: By switching out your chocolate or candies for some fresh fruit, you are telling your brain that you no longer want to load up

- Homemade electrolyte drink can help ease the craving

- Just try to keep yourself busy to take your mind off your cravings or what you think are your cravings

To help curb cravings eat foods that are naturally high in fiber — vegetables, beans and whole grains

CHAPTER 8
WHEN SHOULD I WORKOUT

Working out is the new drug for most people in stressful jobs & has been copied by many who don't even have a stressful life as it can uplift anyone whose feeling depressed or who wants to look good. What type of workout does the average person do during intermittent fasting & what type of workout should you do to combat the many ailments that go with being unfit. Firstly remember that most people think that by working out seven times a week, they will turn themselves into Arnold, but this just isn't the case at all. Latest scientific studies have found that short intensive bursts of exercise will give you the same results as exercising full time.

Smart people are now beginning to see that this is indeed true; these people used to go to the gym several times a week to keep up their physique but now only go three times a week & implement a shorter work out plan. The trick is to follow these programs to the tee & take no rest in between, its takes a while to get used to but once you practice this routine it becomes the second nature to you. You'll then have more time to do other things rather than walk around the gym waiting for the next machine to become available.

The turbulence training program boasts just this; it can give you all the returns in just three days of work out you'd normally need several days to accomplish. This program starts with wide squats, back push up, basic lunge, mountain climbers & jumping jacks to name but a few. Some of the people who tried the above lost up to 26 pounds in under a month, hard to believe isn't is but these guys are the real deal. Almost everyone who took this program lost weight within three weeks & they didn't even go on any diet. That's amazing results, imaging just going to the gym or even staying at home, completing this 40 minute program three days a week & losing weight.

So according to these guys, diets are out the window, you simply don't need to put yourself through all the pain of not being able to eat the things you crave, you just do this intensive work out three times a week & you'll lose the weight. It's an easy decision for most who see this in action, they'll invest in this program because it works & for the small price you'll pay its worth it a thousand fold.

The best way to approach this it to set some goals for yourself, decide now how much weight you want to lose every week, decide on some workout tools like the mini stair stepper to help you along the way, then develop a plan around it. It might also be a good idea to stand in front of a long mirror in your birthday suit & take a photo or two, by doing this you can look back & compare how you looked a few weeks earlier. Many people who use this method say that it gives them an incentive to continue because they can see immediate results

It seems like everyone these days are out to find the best way to get a six-pack, specifically the Intermittent fasting work out. A lower ab work out routine is normally the hardest and most difficult area of the body for people to train and experience definition. So, the first thing people typically turn to is the latest ab machine in the market place. It may be because of all the claims companies make to suck consumers in on an emotional level. It may even come through a lack of knowledge of how to work this area of the body, so they turn to object that makes the most sense. If you sit back and think about it, there have been quite a lot of machines that have made their way into people's home. Of course a lot of the high price machines end up collecting dust in a closet or making their appearance in garage sales every summer. So what's the deal? Here is a lower ab exercise routine that will give you that sharp and dense midsection you have always wanted.

First We Need To Lose The Giggle

I don't care what your trainer says or how well an ab product claims to work, you won't see definition in your midsection if you don't cut back on the calories. This is not rocket science! You can blast your abs to death every day of your life and still not see results. Why? If you are consuming more calories than what you are burning, your belly fat will

still continue to hide those amazing abs you worked so hard to train. The faster you understand this problem, the faster and easier it will be for your abs to "shine." This is why I am a huge fan of combining intermittent fasting with high intensity interval training. Intermittent fasting creates a significant caloric deficit while HIIT burns more calories in the shortest amount of time than traditional cardio. Now that we have established that your diet is more of the culprit than anything, we can move forward. Let's jump right in to the lower ab exercises so when you do lose the fat; your midsection will look like a million bucks.

Work out Routine

1. Hanging Knee Ups
2. Hanging Bent Leg Raises
3. Swinging Side to Side Bent Knee Ups (This will really sculpt the "V" where the hips and lower abs meet.)
4. Planks
5. Hip Bridges/Back Bridges

Note: You will want to do exercises 1&2 for about 15-20 reps with 3-4 sets.

Exercise 3 is performed until you can't lift your knees anymore. At first, you may not be able to do that much. Be consistent and work your way up. Planks are performed for 1 minute with a 30-45 second rest — try this 3-4 times.

Your entire core should be smoked by now! Whatever you do, don't skimp out on the Hip Bridge/Back Bridges. Try a few sets for two minutes. Hip bridges will improve your posture and flexibility immediately. You may even feel a little taller after doing them. You will only need to use this routine 2-3 a week

All these exercises above are a must for maximum ab definition and lower back strength.

Spend your time with this ab routine now so when summer rolls around, you will be prepared for the beach.

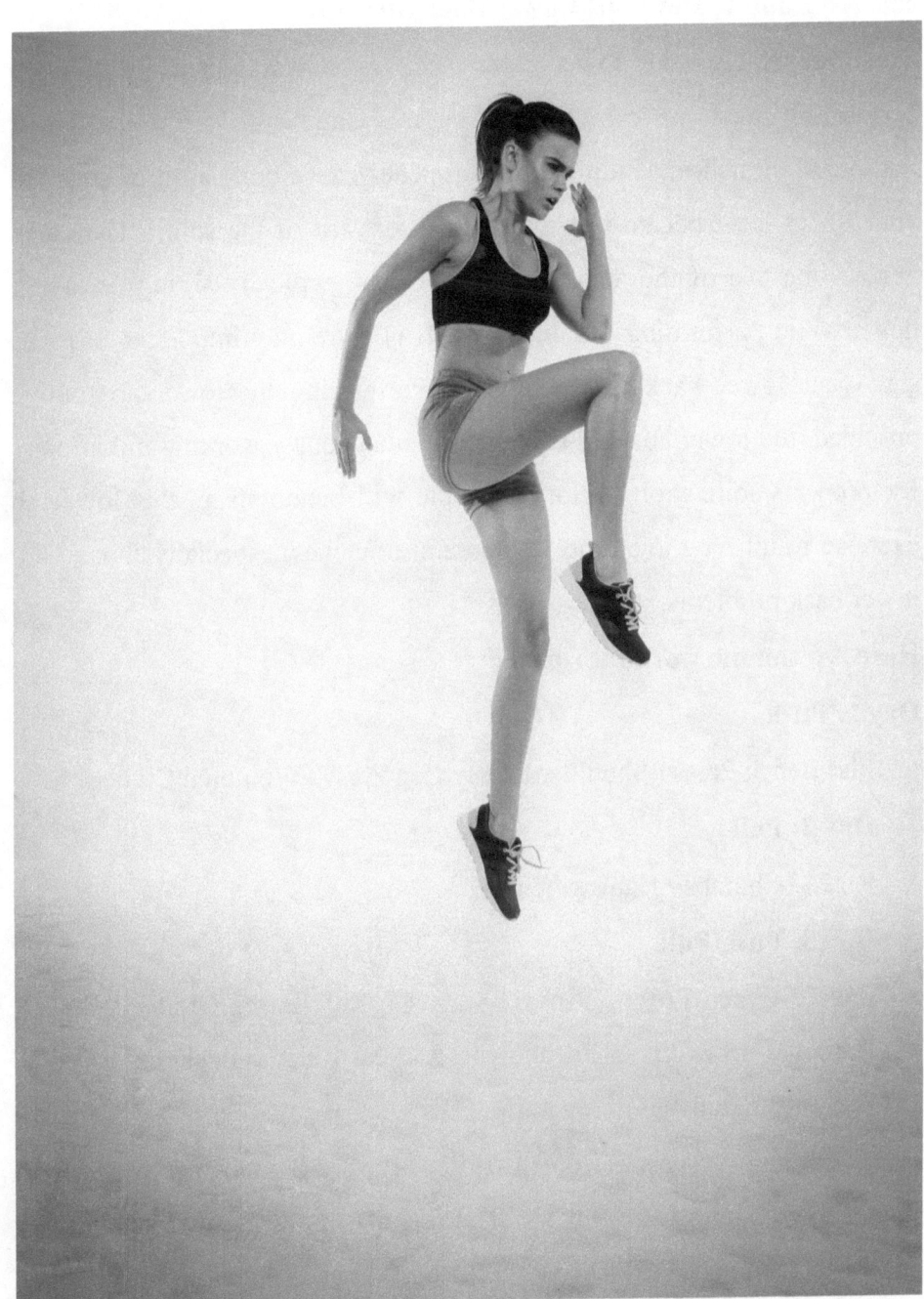

The Ab Routine Develops Lower Back Strength

You may notice your lower back receiving a workout while you are performing these moves. This is a huge reason why I am not a fan of traditional crunches. Traditional ab crunches cause quite a bit of stress to your lower back because of the flexing forward of the spine. They also neglect the use of the spine because you are typically sitting or laying down while performing the exercises. It is extremely important to make sure your lower back is conditioned. Performing the lower ab routine provided, the lower abs and back are simultaneously working in harmony for proper stabilization. A lot of people will benefit from this lower ab exercise routine by avoiding sit ups and crunches, especially those with lower back problems.

Here is a sample workout routine:

Day 1: Push

- Flat Bench Press / Shoulder Press / Leg Press / Weighted Crunches
  Day 2: Pull

- Rows / Chinups / Hamstring Curl
  Day 3: Push/Pull

- Incline Bench Press / Rows / Squats / Calf Raises / Lateral Raise / Barbell Curl / Tricep Pushdown / Lateral Raise / Back Extensions / Weighted Crunches

For maximum fat loss, cardio should be down 2-3 times per week. Start with a five minutes warm up and then begin 10 minutes of High Intensity Interval Training, or HIIT. This works best on an elliptical or a spin bike, instead of a treadmill. You will do this in one minute intervals. Max intensity for one minute followed by a moderate pace for one minute. Repeat until ten minutes are up. After the HIIT session is over, drink some water and rest for five minutes. After your rest, do 30 minutes of Low to Moderate Intensity, Steady State Cardio. A treadmill works great for this.

Intermittent Fasting Diet Weight Training Routine

Weight training is a full body three days routine. Again, exact days don't really matter, but make sure you have a day off in between workouts. You will be working the large muscles only (legs, back, chest) on days 1 and 2 and will add in the smaller muscles arms/calves) on day 3. You will do four sets of 6-8 reps for each large muscle and 2-3 sets of 8-12 for the smaller ones.

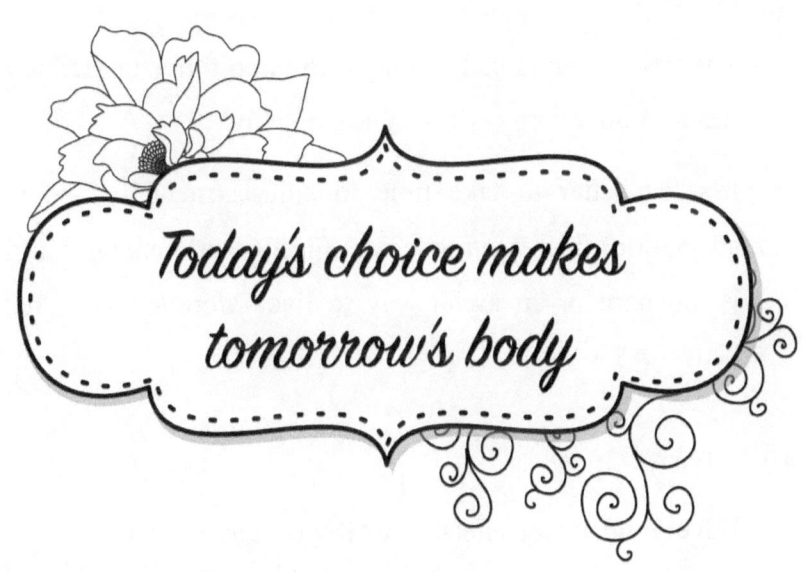

Today's choice makes tomorrow's body

CHAPTER 9
HELP !

Let's get started with some questions about what intermittent fasting is, common mistakes that people make and some problems…

I'm so hungry… What can I do?

- That is TOTALLY normal! Your body is used to burning through glycogen stores for energy. The exhaustion will eventually pass, and your body will become fat-adapted. This means that your body will switch from glycogen stores to your own body fat for energy!

- No need to jump in at 20 hours. Start 12/12, then 16/8, 18/6 and everywhere in between. Ease into it and give your body time to adjust.

- The first few days can be tough. But don't give up. Drink LOTS of water! Your energy will increase quickly.

- It's far better to take time to adjust (mentally and actual fat adaptation) than white-knuckle misery fast, making you think this is too hard or an awful way to live. More/longer is not always better.

I can't lose weight

- Have your doctor check your thyroid, and make sure it's the full panel.

- Maybe try switching up your fasting times. Tricking your body to find out what works for you is best as long as you're still clean fasting, no matter what. Don't give up!
- You should try some 16:8, 18:6, 20:4 fasts, and that varies by day and not week!

Weight gaining

I've been doing the Intermittent Fasting 18:6 for over two weeks and I'm gaining weight. I don't get it.

- 18:6 is a typical maintenance schedule. Longer fasts are the way to go for fat loss.
- Extend your fast by 2 hours and shorten your eating window. Or a 24 hour fast and OMAD (One Meal A Day), and eat until satisfied.
- Keep a tight pair of jeans around; they will tell you more information than the scale.
- Don't weigh yourself so often. It will drive you crazy. So it all works out in the end. Weigh in only once a week or less. The scale will tell you only how much total body mass is being acted upon by gravity. It will not tell you the composition of that mass (lean muscle tissue, fat, bone, water, minerals, etc.)
- Fasted walks, no processed foods, no artificial sweeteners, plenty of good salt, do higher carb eating windows (150-200 carbs) then low carb feeding windows. Focus on nutritionally

dense foods when you are eating. Try to build lean muscle with weight lifting when you are eating.

Fasting insomnia

- *It's time to sleep and you are starving. So much you can't sleep. What do y'all do to get past that? It's annoying!*
- Brush your teeth!
- Drink some water.
- Change your eating window as you find it too difficult to sleep when hungry.
- Try to eat higher fat/lower carbs. It will fill you up more adequately.
- Make sure you end your eating window with protein. Eat enough in your window if you are low on carbs. And, if possible, get to bed before the hunger gets so bad you can't sleep.
- Cup of hot water with a pinch of Himalayan salt.
- Try magnesium supplements.
- Light meditation before bed, the calm app and audio books at bedtime.

Constipation

Constipation is usually caused by a disorder of bowel function rather than a structural problem. Here are some recommendations as you are fasting, which you can do as you also break your fasting:

- Chia gel before bedtime, take 1-2 tsp castor oil diluted in orange juice on an empty stomach, or 1 tsp baking soda in ½ cup warm water.

- Senna leaf tea (Smooth Move tea) before bed.

- Drink some water with sea salt.

- Drink more water

- Adults should consume 25-30 g fiber per day. A lot of people skip on fiber when they start dieting. Don't cut out low carb, high fiber foods! Leafy greens (lettuce, collards, mustard, etc.); broccoli, cauliflower, asparagus, cabbage, and brussel sprouts! Not only will your digestion improve, but you'll feel better, and you'll feel fuller longer.

Diarrhea

- You may want to add in a probiotic and an enzyme to your day about 30 to 40 minutes before opening your window.

- Try less coffee, more water, and break your fast with something small, then give yourself 30 min for a meal. That will help prevent you from overeating, too.

- Break your fast with a glass of metamucil. The fiber will help bulk everything up. After a few weeks, this will pass and you won't need the fiber anymore.

Unhealthy Food Addiction

You eat what you want: unhealthy, too much and junk food included. You don't see any benefit, you don't lose a single pound and you don't want to be careful about what you are eating. Is it useful to continue to fast when you see no benefits whatsoever?

- Even if you can't skip the junk food, try making some of those items you like from scratch, like burgers, noodles, pizzas. You'll find that just by you cooking them with ingredients you can see, it will impact your health for the better. Small steps; you're already fasting so you already have one step down, keep your head up and trust the process. Also, don't be so scale-oriented; focus on how your clothes fit.

- If you don't limit what you eat, but you do pay attention to how many times you eat in your window, that can make a difference. You have naturally grown to want more healthy items. Don't give up, just tweak and see what works for you.

- Fasting also helps us to have appetite correction. For some people, the satiety hormones have been disused/out of whack for so long that it can take months for them to really kick in.

Headaches

I have headaches, what should I do?

- Drink water and sleep enough.

- Break your fast with a cup of bullion for the salt. Just throw a chicken cube in a cup of hot water.

- Try pink salt.

Stretch marks

I'm losing weight, but getting stretch marks. Why?

- You should try to take Collagen.

- Assuming you're not losing weight too quickly, stretch marks are due to stretching your skin further than it's meant to stretch normally.

- Your skin has already been stretched from putting weight on. Now that you're losing it, the skin is retracting, making the existing stretch marks appear more visible.

- Longer fasting will initiate autophagy and your skin will more likely tighten up!

CHAPTER 10
FAQ'S FOR BEGINNERS ABOUT INTERMITTENT FASTING

Vitamines

hat supplements should I be taking?

W A multivitamin, an omega three source, a probiotic, and Vitamin D. I prefer whole food sources over artificial multivitamins. So I would use a greens source as my multivitamin. I use a high quality fish oil or krill oil for my omega three source. An alternative for vegans would be flaxseed oil or hemp oil. As for probiotics, the best source is naturally fermented foods such as miso soup, kimchi, natto, kefir, and sauerkraut. As for supplementation, get one that has more than ten billion active probiotic strains per serving. Vitamin D supplementation is very important for people who don't get one hour of sunlight exposure per day. For instance, if you live in the northeast US, you will need it. People with darker complexions will need more sun exposure than light skinned folks because UV-B rays do not penetrate the skin as far. Therefore, less sunlight is converted to Vitamin D. The latest studies are saying that almost everyone is deficient in Vitamin D.

Protein Supplements

When should I take my protein supplement: before or after a workout?

If you can afford it both. The influx of branch chained amino acids taken before will give you a better performance throughout your workout. The optimal time to take a protein supplement is within 30 minutes of completing your workout for recovery if you are trying to save money.

I have tried all diets …

I have tried all diets and they have failed. What's the easiest way to see results without dieting?

Intermittent fasting may work for you because it's a lifestyle. Research shows that the 18th hour is the "golden hour." This is when you see the most results for the least amount of time. There are different theories on intermittent fasting. Some say the fast starts after your last meal and others say that it starts two or three hours after your last meal due to digestion. Dr. John Fitzgerald wrote an amazing book on intermittent fasting. In it, he gives the easiest way to fast: eat dinner at 6 pm, skip breakfast, and eat lunch at noon.

Immune Function

Does intermittent fasting improves Immune Function (Immune system booster)?

The white blood cells of humans are an effective defense mechanism against pathogens in the body. However, white blood cells are limited by their ability to carry out their defensive function in entering cell and attacking intercellular pathogens. This is because the primary line of defense of these pathogens are lysosomes. Lysosomes through a process known as autophagy, which means self-eating, acts like the garbage disposal of the cell.

Damaged proteins, organelles, viruses, bacteria, and other pathogens are destroyed during autophagy. How long it is before your last meal directly impact lysosomal activities. Are you seeing the connection yet? The function of lysosomes is to control the amount of nutrients that are available to the cells for the organelles to use. A filled stomach suppressed the functions of lysosomes and hence autophagy will not take place. Intermittent fasting allows the cells to undergo autophagy and hence lysosomes can carry out its garbage disposal function. Autophagy is essential in destroying intercellular pathogens by restricting their source of nutrient. A dysfunction in autophagy at the cellular level can lead to all sorts of problem such as certain cancers, speeding up the aging process as well as neurological diseases.

Is it the Right Choice For Me?

Is an Intermittent Fasting Diet the Right Choice For Me? So, does an intermittent fasting lifestyle work when compared to other diets? The answer here is a resounding yes. For example using a 16-hour fast will keep your body burning fat for most of every day! And getting all of your calories during a relatively small eating window stops your body from going into starvation mode and desperately hanging onto body-fat. Compared to a normal reduced calorie diet, this is a huge difference. While any reduced calorie approach will initially lead to fat-loss, your body is an efficient machine and will compensate by slowing down your metabolism (the exact opposite of what you want) and holding onto body fat.

Is an intermittent fasting lifestyle restrictive?

Any diet, by its very nature, involves making better food choices. If someone tries to sell you on the pancake diet, run a mile! Eating rubbish can never be a good choice. However, most diets will have you try to eat clean all the time. this is very hard to do and is directly linked to finding yourself eating 12 doughnuts in one sitting after a couple of weeks of deprivation! Intermittent fasting also involves healthy food choices, but it does give you more wiggle room. It is difficult to eat to much junk in a small eating window after you have already had your healthy food. It does let you eat enough to stop you falling off the wagon however. Perhaps, the real advantage of intermittent fasting is that it can be a lifestyle rather than a short-term approach.

With most diets, even if you do manage to follow it long enough to get results tend to be followed by a rebound that is, a return to poor eating and fat gain. By viewing fasting as a long-term solution, this problem effectively disappears.

Why High Protein, Low Fat, Low Carb?

A couple of reasons;

1. You want to keep calories as low as possible, as easily as possible.

2. Protein plus lots of bulky yet low carb density foods provides the easiest way to feel full, satisfied and happy when cutting calories.

Metabolism

Are low calorie intakes like this necessary for Intermittent Fasting to work? Is Intermittent Fasting, at its core, about calorie restriction in a way that doesn't slow your metabolism and leave you feeling deprived?

- When you eat throughout the day, but in insufficient amounts, you are hungry the whole time and you are fighting that hunger. The body fights back by lowering your metabolism. When you are fasting, particularly once you are acclimated to it, you aren't hungry all day outside your eating window, so you're not fighting your body -- and during your eating window you eat until satiated (again not fighting your body), so it doesn't fight back. The body regulates the metabolic rate based on its perceived fuel.

Insulin resistance

Which fasting regiment is best to solve Insulin resistance?

- LCHF (low-carb high-fat) eating plan, 3 x 36 or 3 x 42 hours per week fast, or Keto.
- Reduce the insulin and your body becomes less resistant to it. Fasting is the quickest way to reduce the levels of insulin in your body. The longer the fasts, the longer the time your cells aren't exposed to insulin, and the quicker the results.

CONCLUSION

What is intermittent fasting and why should you care? Intermittent fasting has become quietly popular in circles where people are striving to come up with ways to reduce caloric intake without harming their workout goals and still allow them to lose weight while strength training.

Intermittent fasting in a nutshell is the practice of short-term fasts, 24 hours in length, once or twice per week. There are variations on that theme, but in general that is the norm. This is done not so much to "cleanse the system" as many would have you believe, though it will to a degree. It's merely a simple and fast way of decreasing caloric intake so you can achieve your weight loss goals without starvation plans or other fad diets. You don't have to be overly concerned about the types of food you consume while you're not fasting, although it should be noted that fasting once or twice per week won't help you reach your goals if you spend the other five or six days stuffing yourself with all manner of junk. A little common sense is called for.

By allowing sensible freedom in your food choices, it relieves a great deal of the anxiety present when it comes to most diets. Many times we feel constrained and restricted, while this approach leaves us able to not only choose what we'd like to consume, but brings balance and sanity back into our diets. Intermittent fasting as a lifestyle will bring about changes that will last a lifetime. Start by taking it slow at first, and learn to listen to what your body is trying to tell you as you go through your first few weeks of this. If you find yourself feeling lethargic or underfed, change it up a bit. Your body will tell you what it needs. (And that usually isn't a monster double cheeseburger!) Many times, especially at first, your body will be going through some withdrawals, and it's important to learn how to differentiate the signals. Also, you need to factor in what effect any workout routines you may be involved in will have on your intermittent fasting plans.

The most important thing to remember about intermittent fasting is that it is not merely a diet plan, but a lifestyle, worthy of consideration along those lines. In order to get the best results possible from this type of plan, you need to befriend it. Your fasting should be something that you look forward to, as you most certainly will after you start reaping some of the benefits of this

Intermittent Fasting Lifestyle. Making this type of plan fit into your life is key to making a lifetime of good eating and healthy living possible. There are a lot of inherent freedoms built into a diet plan like this, and while that can backfire on you if you're not careful, it can also enable lasting success. Look into what intermittent fasting can do for you!

WHO SHOULDN'T USE INTERMITTENT FASTING

There are specific circumstances under which intermittent fasting isn't ideal or shouldn't be used. While it is an effective tool, everyone's biochemistry is different and can vary at different stages or times in your life.

You should NOT use intermittent fasting if you are:

- Suffering from adrenal fatigue. **Adrenal fatigue** can occur when you are under a lot of intense stress, have suffered an infection or illness, or are severely sleep-deprived. Adrenal fatigue makes you very tired, and it affects the way you metabolize your food.

- **Pregnant or nursing:** you should be eating regularly to sustain the increased caloric needs of growing baby and milk production.

- **Have or are recovering from an eating disorder:** It's important to have and maintain a healthy relationship with food. Please seek professional help if you have an eating disorder. And, If you are recovering from an eating disorder or have struggled with eating disorders in the past, please do not use intermittent fasting as a weight-loss tool.

- **Are a child:** Children are growing while they sleep and need a good quality breakfast to replenish their spent energy. An ideal should not include fruit juice or grains, but rather protein and vegetables like a Green Monster Frittata or boiled eggs, meat, and vegetables.

Consult your healthcare professional prior to beginning a fast if you have any condition you are concerned will be negatively affected by a change in diet.

Because of the female hormone cycle, intermittent fasting may not be as effective for some women. However, other women find it to be an incredibly useful tool either on a regular basis or during specific times when they want to tone up quickly.

Intermittent fasting weight loss lifestyle is radically different from most weight loss programs being promoted in the market. However, its ideas are scientifically sound when it comes to losing weight. You should give this program a go if you are serious about weight loss.

After knowing **The Intermittent Fasting: How to Live Fit, Lose Weight fast and Stay Young. Inspiring Beginner's Guide**, it is advisable to work towards your goals of losing weight for healthy life draw a plan of your goals and work towards it.

As Cheryl Strayed once said, "It's up to you to make your life. Take what you have and stack it up like a tower of teetering blocks. Build your dream around that."

Thanks for reading. I hope you enjoyed this book.

WANT FREE GOODIES ABOUT IF ?!

Just email me at

my.healthy.life.plans@gmail.com

title the email « IF Free Gift »

and let me know that you purchased

The Intermittent Fasting Beginner's Guide

and I'll send you something fun!

PROGRESS

I Feel More Connected With Myself

_____

_____

_____

_____

_____

_____

I'm doing more exercice

_____

_____

_____

_____

_____

I'm eating more healthier

_____

_____

_____

_____

_____

Progress Chart

PROGRESS CHART						
Date	Weight	L/R Arm	L/R Leg	Chest	Waist	Hip

WEEKLY WEIGHT LOSS TRACKER

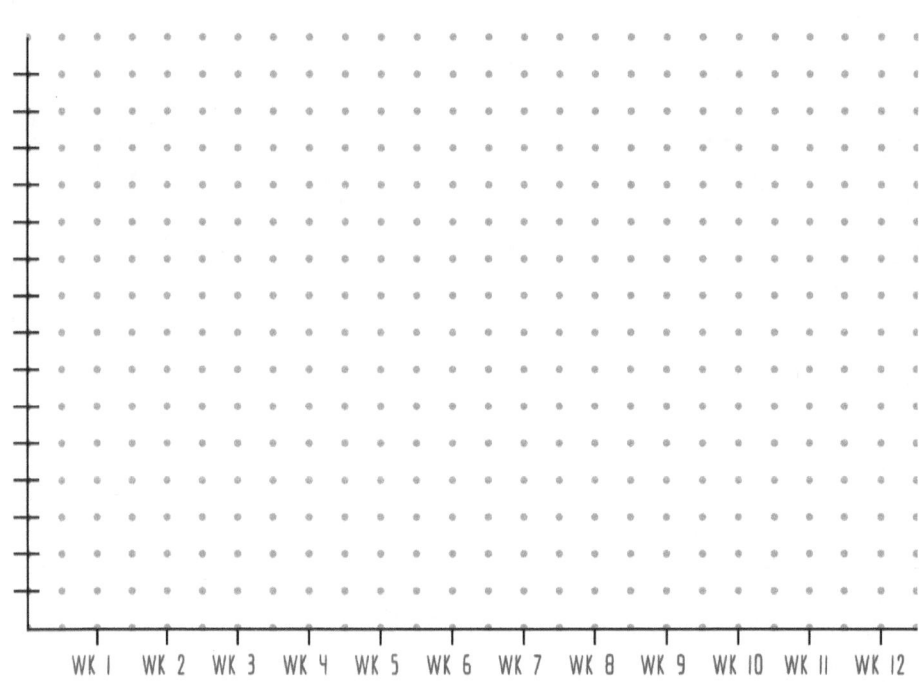

WK 1   WK 2   WK 3   WK 4   WK 5   WK 6   WK 7   WK 8   WK 9   WK 10   WK 11   WK 12

WEEKLY WEIGHT LOSS TRACKER

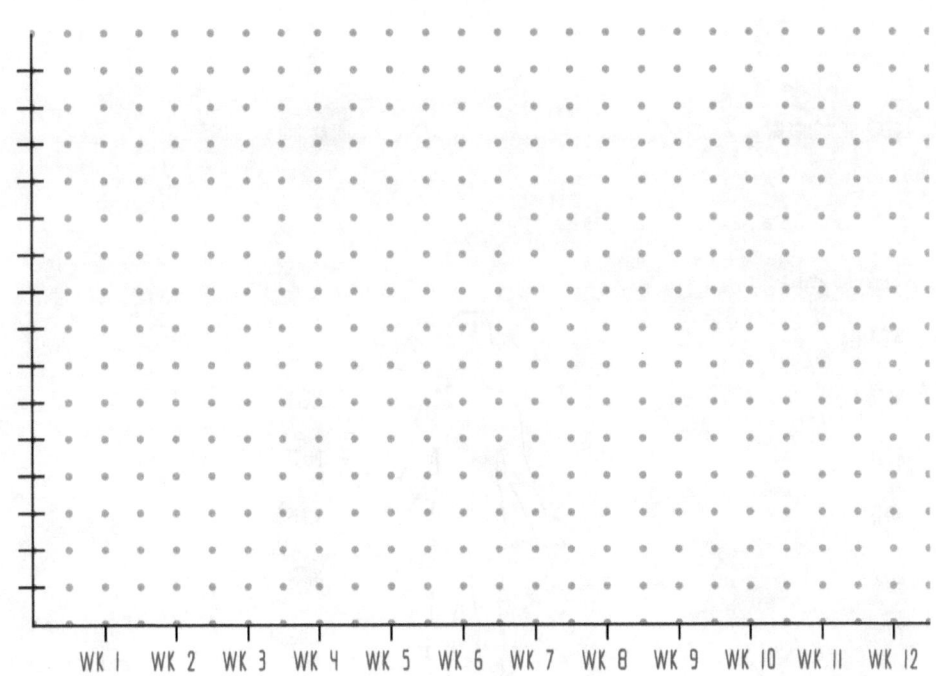

WK 1   WK 2   WK 3   WK 4   WK 5   WK 6   WK 7   WK 8   WK 9   WK 10   WK 11   WK 12

BEFORE & AFTER

YOUR
[PICTURE HERE]
3.1 X 3.1 INCH / 8 X 8CM

YOUR
[PICTURE HERE]
3.1 X 3.1 INCH / 8 X 8CM

AREAS OF CONCERN

IDEAL BODY / SHAPE

STARTING DATE:

END DATE:

WEIGHT:

NECK:

NECK:

BUST:

BUST:

WAIST:

WAIST:

HIPS:

HIPS:

THIGH:

THIGH:

CALF:

CALF:

NOTES:

NOTES:

110

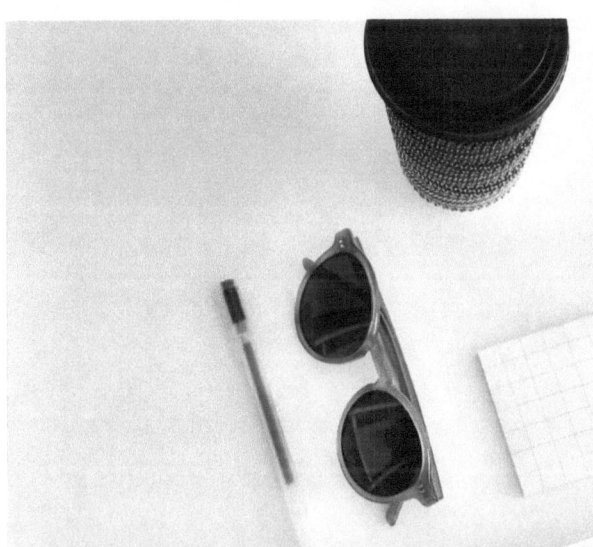

Change your life
today.

Don't gamble
on the future,
act now,
without delay.

Simone de Beauvoir